SURVIVORS: LIVING WITH CANCER

Books by Robert L. Shook

Survivors: Living with Cancer
The Book of Why
The Shaklee Story
The Chief Executive Officers
The Real Estate People
The Entrepreneurs
Ten Greatest Salespersons
Why Didn't I Think of That?
Winning Images
Successful Telephone Selling in the '80s
  (with Martin D. Shafiroff)
How to Be the Complete Professional Salesman
  (with Herbert Shook)
Total Commitment
  (with Ronald Bingamen)

Survivors:
LIVING WITH CANCER

Portraits of Twelve Inspiring People

ROBERT L. SHOOK

HARPER & ROW, PUBLISHERS, New York
Cambridge, Philadelphia, San Francisco, London
1817   Mexico City, São Paulo, Sydney

FIRST EDITION

Designer: Sidney Feinberg

Library of Congress Cataloging in Publication Data

Shook, Robert L., 1938–
    Survivors, living with cancer.

    1. Cancer—Patients—United States—Biography.
I. Title.
RC265.5.S56   1983   362.1'96994'00922 [B]   83–47544
ISBN 0–06–015204–4

83 84 85 86 87 10 9 8 7 6 5 4 3 2 1

TO BOBBIE
With all my love

CONTENTS

ACKNOWLEDGMENTS

There are many people who have directly or indirectly contributed to this book. First and foremost, my publisher Irv Levey deserves credit for encouraging me to write this book. I am also grateful to him for doing an outstanding job editing the manuscript. I also thank Daniel Bial, Irv's assistant.

I also wish to acknowledge Mary Kay Ash, Dr. Sidney Black, Dr. William Cahan, Jenny Guy, Dr. Jerry Guy, Dr. David Leichtman, Dr. Bruce Meyer, Ronna Romney, Dr. Sidney Salk, Lis Smith, Stephanie Simonton, Jack Wilder, Ursula Wolk, and Al Zuckerman.

INTRODUCTION

In the fall of 1976 we discovered that my wife had cancer. Our family nearly fell apart. Bobbie was young—in her early thirties—beautiful, and athletic. We listened in disbelief as the doctor described the seriousness of her cancer. I kept thinking this wasn't really happening. He couldn't be talking about Bobbie Shook. That was impossible. She wasn't sick—she looked the "picture of health," and she felt fine! But, of course, it was real life—not a horrible nightmare from which we'd awaken. It was a waking nightmare that lasted a long, long time.

For the past seven years, it seems as though we've been on a runaway roller coaster. First the diagnosis of cancer and the operation. Then remission, and we thought Bobbie was healthy again. We had actually stopped worrying about cancer when it was diagnosed again. The recurrence was at least as frightening as the original diagnosis. Bobbie had another operation and got better again, and once again we thought the cancer was completely gone. Then an X ray taken during a regular physical showed it was back. Bobbie felt wonderful—but they said she was terribly sick, and must take chemotherapy. The chemotherapy did make her very sick, but we feel it saved her life. She had another remission. Eventually, however, she had another recurrence. Bobbie has gone through this cycle several times.

A number of my books have been about successful people, and one thing I'm certain of—success begets success. So I started looking for books about cancer patients who had survived. I wanted to show Bobbie that not everybody who gets cancer dies from it. I wanted to convince our family—and myself— that Bobbie would get well again. But I couldn't find any books that were really helpful, so I began phoning cancer specialists all over the country. "I'm looking for cancer survivors," I said. "I want to hear their stories." I explained my reasons, of course, but the doctors were understandably reluctant to give their patients' names and addresses. Finally I said, "Look, I'm thinking of writing a book about them—a book that will help and inspire thousands of discouraged, frightened cancer patients and their families." Then I got the support I needed from the doctors. The names poured in. It was incredible to find out that there was no dearth of cancer survivors—they were everywhere!

Getting to know these survivors gave Bobbie and our family hope. Their success showed us that cancer could be overcome. If they could do it, she could, too. The people in this book have maintained hope despite setbacks and discouraging times. Like Bobbie, many of them have had periods of good health broken by the devastating news of recurrence. Even patients who ultimately get well often go through this roller-coaster ride.

The subjects in this book participated in their recoveries in various ways, but all chose traditional medical treatment. I selected only survivors who had worked with established treatment because I wanted this book to be about people, not about controversial treatment plans.

The more I learned, writing this book, the more my fear of cancer diminished. The disease doesn't deserve the stigma associated with it; a diagnosis of cancer is not an automatic death sentence.

As *Living with Cancer* goes to press, we do not know the final outcome of Bobbie's illness. She appears to be fine. She still has cancer, but it's quiet now, and we're enjoying every minute of her wellness. We'd like to believe that she won't have any more bouts with this dreaded disease. At least we know that there is hope that she will live a long and healthy life as other cancer patients have.

SURVIVORS: LIVING WITH CANCER

1

JAY WEINBERG

"I don't like the looks of that mole on your back," the dermatologist told Jay. "I suggest you talk to your family doctor about having it removed."

Jay Weinberg had made the appointment only to discuss a minor skin rash. Nothing in the doctor's manner led him to become alarmed about the mole. Still, he did see his family doctor, and relayed the dermatologist's concern.

"Let's leave it alone," the general practitioner said. "We'll just watch it."

"And that's what we did. We just watched it for two years."

When his family doctor retired, Jay went to another physician for his routine annual checkup. This time he had a complaint—some muscle stiffness in his left arm. He wasn't seriously concerned, however; a fifty-six-year-old man who insisted on playing tennis three times a week had to expect a little soreness. Jay's serenity quickly vanished, though, for within minutes the new doctor had located a lump the size of a ping-pong ball under Jay's left arm.

"A lump? What does that mean?" Jay asked.

"I don't know yet. We should probably put you in the hospital and remove it." Jay decided to get a second opinion.

The second doctor studied the lump and then asked, "How long have you had this mole on your back?"

Jay explained, as the doctor frowned.

"The lump and the mole may be related," the doctor said finally. "They've got to be removed."

On March 23, 1974, Jay was admitted to the local hospital for a simple procedure; he expected to be operated on one day and go home the next. The removal of the lump was preceded by a biopsy of the mole. Jay was given sedation, and the operating room was prepared for surgery.

When the ominous report arrived, Jay was too sedated to understand; the surgeon talked to his wife, Marian, instead. The biopsy showed malignancy. The operation would have to be far more extensive than they had planned.

Marian, knowing her husband was in no position to protect himself, asked the surgeon, "When was the last time you did an operation like this?"

"Five years ago."

"I'm terribly sorry," Marian said, "but I'm taking my husband out of here. I want him someplace where they've done five operations like this—yesterday."

Jay was still under the effects of the sedation and unaware of what was going on. Marian escorted him out of the hospital, and drove him home. While Jay dozed on the couch, she called the family physician, and asked him to arrange to have Jay treated at Memorial Sloan-Kettering Cancer Center in New York City. "I realize now that I did all the right things, but I was scared out of my mind. When Jay woke up, I told him calmly what I had arranged. I didn't think it would do him any good to see how I did feel—but I didn't feel calm."

The following Monday Jay had an appointment at Memorial Sloan-Kettering with Dr. Man He Shiu. After examining the biopsy slides and giving Jay a thorough physical, Dr. Shiu

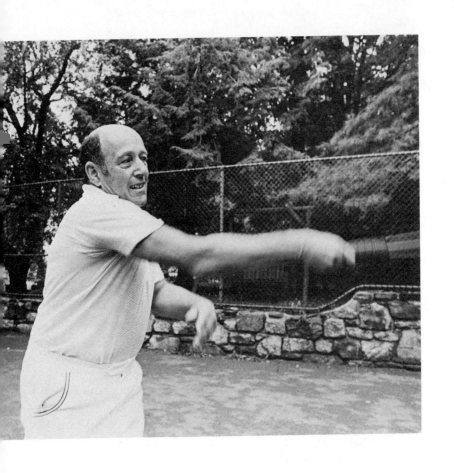

JAY WEINBERG

told Jay and Marian the matter-of-fact verdict: "Malignant melanoma. This is a very capricious type of cancer—it can pop up anywhere in your body. Frankly, we know very little about this type of cancer, except that we have to operate.

"As for your particular situation, Mr. Weinberg," Dr. Shiu continued, "it is very serious, we do not know to what extent. We know the mole was malignant and the lump under your arm has appeared as a result. We do not know how much further it has spread. It will be several days until we have a hospital bed for you. Meanwhile, I suggest you go home and get your affairs in order."

In one dizzying day Jay Weinberg had changed from a man with a lump and a little mole to a man confronting death. He could hardly absorb it, and was swept by one reaction after another.

"I was scared, and I was angry," he says, "angry because it wasn't *fair*. I'd always been in good health, there was no history of cancer in my family, and I'd never smoked. I thought, 'Why me? I'm a healthy guy, I've got a great life. Why me?'

"I also felt helpless, because I knew nothing about this cancer, and at the moment I didn't have anyone to turn to except Dr. Shiu. He was a stranger to me, and like many surgeons, he seemed cold and tough. He inspired a lot of confidence, though. I could tell that he was good. I felt it in his touch when he examined me; I sensed that he knew what he was doing. So, in the middle of all my other emotions, at least I did have confidence in my surgeon."

During the nerve-wracking week before his admission to Memorial Hospital, Jay got his affairs in order. "But I *never* accepted the possibility that I could die," he says emphatically. "I wouldn't accept it. Nothing was going to wipe me out at that point in my life, because I had too many things to do. I wasn't ready to leave my family."

He sighs and adds, "But Dr. Shiu was right, of course. So I

did prepare everything—my will was in order, my finances arranged properly, my desk clean. I was prepared for the worst . . . but I never accepted the idea that it could actually happen to me."

One major area Jay didn't have to worry about was the Avis Rent A Car franchise in southern Westchester, New York, which he had owned for over twenty years. His son, Jim, now in his late twenties, had been working with Jay in the business for some time. Now, as he prepared to enter Memorial Hospital, Jay decided the timing was right to make a major change. He told Jim, "Okay, the time has come for you to be the boss. Now I'm the second in command."

On April 1, Jay Weinberg walked into Memorial Hospital for an operation that might save his life. As he was about to enter the building, he stopped abruptly, and Marian had to come back for him.

"Must be an April Fools' Day joke," he said, looking around. "But I don't see anybody." He bent and picked up the dollar bill under his toe. "This is a good omen," he told Marian, his eyes lighting up. "You know what? This really gives me hope." He meant it. That dollar bill became a symbol of good luck, and today it is framed and hangs on Jay's bedroom wall.

It was not easy to keep up spirits during the six days of preliminary testing in the hospital. Like many patients, Jay visualized the cancer spreading rapidly throughout his body. "Each second that ticks away is precious time lost," he thought. Before he knew that there was a lump under his arm, Jay had felt only minor discomfort in that arm. Now that he knew it was there, and it was cancer, he couldn't stop thinking about it. "It seemed to come alive," he says, "and it felt bigger and bigger every day. I couldn't understand why they weren't operating right *now*. But I learned that it's not that urgent to operate; what is urgent is to take a good look at what's there—that's the preliminary test. First they look; then they operate. That's a lot better than operating first and looking later.

"It shook me up when they asked me to sign releases before the operation. I said, 'What is *this* about?' The doctor explained that while he was operating, he had to have the freedom to take action, quickly and decisively. He had to be able to do what should be done. That made sense; I signed the releases.

"I wasn't really afraid of dying," Jay continues, "and I had learned enough not to be afraid of suffering. With modern chemistry, pain is a secondary concern. What *did* scare me was the possibility that I might not be able to function normally after the operation. I've always been an active person, and I hated the thought of becoming a burden to my wife and family."

During his tests, Jay continually asked questions, and when he didn't get clear answers, he pushed for them. He explains, "They didn't volunteer information. It's not that the doctors were callous—they just didn't have the time. But I had so many questions, I just kept firing away. I believe patients should do that; they should know everything, as much as they can absorb. I asked about everything: 'How long will this take?' 'When am I going to get out?' 'How serious is it?' 'How long before we see the end results of this?' 'What are my options?' 'What are the percentages? The chances?'"

Jay knew that his situation was very serious and his life was in jeopardy. He asked, "Have you ever saved *anyone* with this kind of cancer?"

"Of course," Dr. Shiu said firmly. Jay was afraid to press for more specific information, and the doctor didn't volunteer to tell Jay that his chances for long-term survival were remote.

On April 8, after the operation, Marian asked Dr. Shiu, "Did you get everything you wanted?" He answered, "Yes."

"What are my chances of a normal life now?" Jay asked the next day.

"Good. Your chances are good."

"My daughter Joan is getting married May 11. Will I be able to attend?"

"You may well be able to walk her down the aisle."

The surgeon had removed all the lymph nodes under Jay's left arm, as well as a large area of skin surrounding the malignant mole. The toughest part of the recovery for Jay was enduring the discomfort of the extensive skin grafts taken from his leg and placed on his back. Doing his best to ignore the pain, he was up and walking the day after the surgery. On the third day he decided he would have a goal; he would walk a mile a day. But how could he know he had walked a mile? Jay measured one of the square tiles that paved the long corridors of the hospital, and calculated that if he walked around his floor eleven times, he would walk exactly one mile. His first goal was simply to make that mile, however long it might take.

From then on, the short, bald man wearing a white hospital gown under a blue bathrobe could be seen walking the halls, his expression determined but cheerful. His progress was slow, since he paused to say hello to everyone he met. He was so friendly that one nurse routinely kidded, "You running for mayor of New York, Jay?"

The walking was initially exhausting. To keep himself busy while he rested up, Jay got on the telephone and investigated a vacation dream—a raft trip down a river in Idaho. With Marian insisting, "Jay, you're *crazy*, you'll never be well enough to do that this summer," he nevertheless sent in an application and deposit for the two of them.

Jay was taking the right approach—overcoming the boredom that accompanies any hospital stay. When books and games weren't enough to occupy him, Jay talked to other patients, some of whom were unable to get out and walk as he was.

"Actually," he says, "I didn't realize it, but I was sometimes giving them pep talks. It was therapeutic for them and for me, and I was probably the chief beneficiary. I'd go in, listen to what they had to say, describe some of the problems I'd had, offer some encouragement. That really puts things in perspective, because there's always somebody in the hospital worse off than you are." Many of the forty patients on Jay's floor were being treated for similar problems, melanomas and skin cancers. Since Memorial is a specialized cancer hospital, each of its eighteen floors is devoted to a certain type of cancer, and all medical personnel on each floor become specialists. "This is one benefit of a center," Jay says. "Another is that you're together with patients who have the same illness, so you can encourage one another. Sometimes that's not so easy."

Jay had to deal with the impending death of his roommate. The man had been friendly with Jay, but avoided the subject of dying, even though he was desperately ill. "It did bother me to be in this atmosphere," Jay admits soberly. "But I was rooting for him, and I thought if I asked for a room change I'd be deserting a friend."

As his roommate's condition grew worse, there were more visits to the room by doctors and nurses, particularly at night, and Jay found it harder and harder to sleep. Finally one night, when his roommate required constant attention, Jay asked to be given a bed in another room, just for the night. He was refused. Nevertheless, he found an empty room down the hall, climbed into the bed, and went to sleep—until he rolled over and hit the call button. The nurse who answered the signal told him in no uncertain terms to go to his room.

"Now, there I was," Jay says with a shrug, "a fifty-six-year-old guy getting hell for sneaking out to find a place to sleep!" He agreed to return to his room, then slipped away to an empty lounge on the other side of the floor. There he slept undisturbed. When he returned to his room in the early morning, it was empty; his roommate had died.

For Jay, as for every cancer patient, maintaining a positive, outgoing attitude was essential. He was immeasurably helped by family members and friends who understood his need to be part of "the real world out there." During his hospital stay, his son, Jim, called frequently to talk business. "He didn't bug me with day-to-day details," Jay explains, "but we did talk about everything major. I also got calls from the chairman of the Advertising and Policy Committee for the Avis franchisees—I'm one of the people elected to that board. The chairman called just to keep me posted. I appreciated those calls. They made me feel I wasn't being left out."

Jay received invaluable support from his family. Marian visited daily, Jim visited when he could, and daughters Ann and Joan took turns flying in from the West Coast. Although flying together would have been more pleasant, they reasoned that they'd get more mileage out of separate visits. "When I learned, shortly after the operation, that Ann would be flying in, I was determined to be up and walking. I wanted her to be greeted by her strong father, not someone weak and sickly. Ego, I guess. Anyway, that helped motivate me to keep on walking the halls."

Jay was excited about Joan's wedding, and Marian involved him in as many details as possible. Since Jay could not go shopping for a new suit for the event, Marian brought one from Saks Fifth Avenue, and had their fitter come to the hospital to make the alterations. Realizing that the fitter was on his own time, the Weinbergs tried to pay him—but he insisted that he was glad to help Jay out, and refused to accept even cab fare.

Marian, too, bought a new dress for the wedding, and brought it to the hospital to show Jay. Upon his urging, she agreed to model it for him. Just as she was pulling her dress off over her head, the door opened and in walked Dr. Shiu.

"Excuse me," he said, and left the room.

Jay called him back to explain. "After all, it was only four days after my operation. But I'm not sure he ever did believe my story. From that time on, he always called me 'Tiger.'"

Released from the hospital on April 24, Jay received ongoing treatment as an outpatient. Meanwhile, he helped with plans for the wedding, including engineering the assembly of the homemade four-tiered cake. The wedding took place in nearby Greenwich, Connecticut, as planned, and everything went smoothly. Jay was indeed able to walk Joan down the aisle and give her away.

By midsummer Jay was back at work, and was also working diligently on his tennis game. Every two weeks he visited Memorial for follow-up tests and examination by Dr. Shiu. Then, about three months after the operation, the routine chest X ray showed a spot on Jay's lung. The cancer had metastasized.

This time, Dr. Shiu explained, the operation would be performed by another Memorial doctor, William Cahan, who specialized in thoracic surgery. Dr. Cahan, who had an excellent reputation, couldn't schedule the operation until three weeks later, so Jay and Marian decided to take a vacation at Lake Placid. Jay had recently purchased an Avis franchise there, and while on vacation he talked often about how exciting it was going to be to come back for the Winter Olympics in 1980—six years away.

"Eternal optimism," Marian says with a smile. "Frankly, I thought he was out of his *mind*. Here we were, waiting for this lung surgery, and I was a nervous wreck, and he was talking about how good business was going to be during the Olympics!"

Jay, of course, knew that the metastasis to the lung was a bad sign, as was the quickness of the recurrence. He couldn't help reflecting on the first sign of cancer he'd had, the mole on his back, discovered in 1972. What if it had been removed then and there? Would he have developed cancer at all?

Searching for causes, since he himself did not smoke and there was no history of cancer in his family, Jay heard a theory that cancer can begin after a traumatic experience causes the breakdown of the immune system, making the individual susceptible to disease. Jay remembered the anguish when his son, Jim, had been seriously wounded in Vietnam. "This was the only trauma I could think of," he says. "Could be. But I don't really believe this theory. We know that some people are genetically more susceptible to cancer. So anybody can get it—rich or poor, young or old.

"But whoever you are, you have to help yourself in this situation. I believe in God, but not in a formal religion. I didn't pray before I got cancer, and I didn't pray after. Although I believe in Him, I don't think God alone helps you out of this kind of situation. You have to help yourself, too."

As Dr. Shiu had predicted, Dr. Cahan told the Weinbergs another operation was necessary. This one would require removal of one of the two lobes of Jay's left lung. Because of the shadow on the lung, as well as the fact of a pre-existing cancer, Dr. Cahan believed the operation was definitely called for. But he also told the Weinbergs it was, at best, a gamble. "There's no guarantee that this is a cure," he explained. "It simply gives you a chance."

Dr. Cahan later commented on Jay's solitary metastasis. "Scientists wonder about this phenomenon. After all, they reason, many cancer cells are cast into the circulation. Why should only one take root and grow? This does not happen often but is probably an expression of the host/cancer relationship, and at this time, it's a scientific mystery."

There were people who thought Jay was foolish to undergo additional major surgery, since his type of cancer would probably spread again soon thereafter. "I believed that they were right, but it was the only alternative to doing nothing at all. That made it my preferred option."

When Jay checked into Memorial Hospital in September 1974, he remembered the long days of preliminary testing before his first operation five months ago. Determined to make the most of the time he had, he took Marian and two friends out to dinner. He laughs, recalling what happened. "While we were out, Dr. Cahan came in to see me. Well, I had been out on pass from the hospital, so they told him where I was, and he was concerned—because I was scheduled for surgery at 8:00 in the morning."

When Jay sailed in at 9:00 that night, the nurses promptly put him to bed. Unfortunately, in the confusion nobody prepped him for the operation. "The next morning," Jay says, "they sedated me, put me on the cart, took me downstairs, and rolled me onto the operating table to wait for my chest surgery. The only trouble was, I'm a very hairy guy, and they hadn't shaved my chest. In walked Dr. Cahan, ready to operate, and he took one look at me and roared, "Why isn't he prepped? Get him ready!'"

The surgery went smoothly, and Jay had less discomfort following this operation than he'd had after his first surgery. "It was a good feeling to know that I had everything going for me," Jay says with a smile. "I knew I had a top surgeon, and I was in one of the great cancer centers of the world. That was very reassuring."

Pausing briefly, he adds, "I've heard some people say they're afraid they wouldn't get the same personal attention in a cancer center that they get back home in a local hospital. I suppose they want the doctor to hold their hands, to give them love and affection. Well, some doctors at cancer centers may appear cold and removed at first, but I think this is a protective device; they shield themselves because they're working with the most advanced and complicated cases. But I found that they were very dedicated people who obviously cared a great deal about their patients.

"Your local doctor might be more personally involved initially, especially if he's been on your case for a longer period of time. But if you stick with only local doctors and local hospitals, you may not receive the best care. There are twenty-one cancer centers in this country, and if your case is serious, that's where you should be. Medical teams at these centers do nothing but deal with specific types of cancer. They're good—they're highly trained, and they're experienced. They might not hold your hand. So what? If you want someone to hold your hand, get someone else—but not your doctor."

Jay's immediate confidence in Bill Cahan was based not only on the surgeon's reputation, but on his manner. After the lung operation, Dr. Cahan appeared in Jay's room to say simply, "You're okay."

"He exudes confidence," Jay says. "He said it so decisively that I was *sure* I was okay."

While he was recovering, Jay again set a goal: Avis was holding a convention in Vancouver the next month; he and Marian would be there. He resumed his long walks through the halls of Memorial Hospital until he again reached a mile a day. Meanwhile he periodically reminded Dr. Cahan of his determination to be released for the convention.

In late September Jay signed out of the hospital, and in October he and Marian flew to Vancouver. He was still shaky, and they spent most of their time in their room, looking out at seagulls and resting, with Marian tending his bandages as necessary. "Still," she says, "the trip was great—it did wonders for his attitude. I know it had a lot to do with getting him back on his feet." The trip down the Selway River had to be postponed, but the following summer the couple did take that vacation together.

After the Vancouver trip was over, Jay began the toughest part of his recovery program—an experimental immunization program which Dr. Cahan recommended. "The only thing we can do now is try this program," the doctor had explained. "We've done all we know how to with conventional cancer treatment. Now you either do nothing, or you enter this program, where you'll get injections that we believe may mobilize your immune system to fight the cancer cells. It's a tough decision—and it's up to you."

Faced again with a choice of doing something or doing nothing, Jay chose to do something.

The program, administered by another team of specialists, headed by Carl Pinsky, was not a simple one. For most of November 1974 Jay was an inpatient at Memorial Hospital, going home only on weekends. Each morning, Monday through Friday, he was given an intravenous injection. Following this, he endured a daylong bout with chills and fever. "First I'd get freezing cold," he says, "as if I were on a ski lift, and it was 20 degrees below zero, and I didn't have any clothes on. Then, two or three hours later, my temperature would start to climb. It would go up to 103, then 104, and even close to 105. Finally that would break. By about 6:00 at night I'd feel pretty decent again, and I'd have a good supper. Then the next morning the nurses would come in and raise the dosage. The point of that was always to give me the maximum dose I could take, on the theory that they could determine the maximum dosage to boost my immunization system. The next day I'd get that big injection, and the whole procedure would start all over again.

"I'm a pretty even-tempered fellow," Jay says, "but I didn't like it when those doctors would come around with that question, 'How do you feel today?' I mean, it was pretty obvious how I felt. I'd look at them and say, 'Why don't *you* try a shot of this and see how *you* feel?'"

The month as an inpatient receiving the experimental treatments was the worst part of Jay's entire illness. As the procedure went on, he became depressed. "I had to face that

awful treatment every morning, and it lasted the whole day,"
he says with a grimace. "I was really down. Once I even told
Marian, 'Don't come in tomorrow. I don't want to see anyone.' I just wanted to be alone. When you're feeling that
rotten, it's hard to be sociable. You have to suffer alone. I
don't think anyone wants to have other people around during
those times. You just want to moan a little, I guess, in your
own way.

"There were times when the nurses would come in and I'd
feel like telling them to go away, because I didn't want to go
through with it. But I counted the days. After a while there
were only three weeks to go, and then only two weeks to go,
and then only one. I felt a lot better when I could see the light
at the end of the tunnel."

Enduring the experimental treatments was nerve-wracking
for Jay because there was no way of knowing whether it
would all be worthwhile or not. Nobody could tell him, "Do
this for the next four weeks, and everything will go away."
All he could do was hope that his decision to be a guinea pig
was the best decision in the first place.

By Thanksgiving Day, the worst was over and Jay was released from the hospital. The permanent lock in his arm,
where the IV had been hooked up every day, was removed.
For the next three years he would stay with the program; but
the follow-up injections were subcutaneous, and the side effects much milder. At first Jay received weekly shots as an
outpatient at Memorial Hospital. Although the injection took
only a few minutes, the process entailed three hours of driv-
ing time and a long waiting period between the shot and the
routine examination that followed. Jay used the waiting period to wander back to his old floor and "make the rounds" of
both old friends and new acquaintances. He found some people in need of a good listener; others wanted to hear about his
own problems as a patient. Since he was active and enjoying
life, talking to him was inspirational for many patients.

After three months of outpatient treatments Jay was no longer reacting with chills and fever; now he experienced only a slight chill of short duration after each shot. The easier the treatment became, the more irritated he was over the loss of a full day to get the shot.

"This is ridiculous," he told the hospital staff. "Diabetics give themselves injections like this—why can't I?"

"Nobody's ever done that."

"Then let's get started."

The staff taught Jay to administer the shots to himself. After the first one, he found it easy. When he discovered that other patients in the program were still coming to the hospital for their injections, he wrote out a protocol so that they, too, could give themselves shots at home if they wanted to.

To this day, sections of Jay's tumor are being kept alive in a Sloan-Kettering laboratory; samples of his blood are still killing the tumor—which seems to indicate that he has developed an immunity to the kind of cancer he had. A team of researchers headed by Dr. Philip Livingston is working in this area. After three years, Jay was taken off the program. "Don't you think I was a little nervous then?" he asks. "It was like, 'You're on your own now!'"

Today, however, periodic physicals reveal no signs of cancer at all. The immunization program may be working for Jay, although for some patients it did not; there are not yet enough data to determine whether the treatment can be considered effective overall. Jay believes it has probably saved his life. "And this kind of treatment would not have been available anywhere other than a cancer center," he emphasizes. "I'm very thankful I went to Memorial Sloan-Kettering." It must be noted, however, that there have also been patients with melanoma metastases to the lung who are long-term survivors and *never* took part in an immunization program.

Today, Jay will affirm, his life is better as a result of his bout with cancer. Always an avid tennis player and skier, he has added swimming to his daily routine. Over their backyard pool, the Weinbergs had an air bubble installed, so that Jay can swim his one third of a mile every morning before going to work.

The swimming, intended to strengthen the remaining lobes of Jay's lungs, has also been good for his heart and general muscle tone and endurance—to such an extent that his tennis game is as good as ever. Always a strong player, Jay became confident enough after his second surgery to challenge Dr. Cahan, also a tennis enthusiast, to a game one day.

"It's one thing to advise your patient to increase his activities after surgery," says Bill Cahan with a smile. "It's another to face him across the net. The first time we played, I had very mixed feelings. On the one hand, I was concerned about exhausting Jay with my drop shots, and I also held back from hitting the ball too hard. On the other hand, I suddenly discovered I was losing at an alarming rate. Then I became much more interested in winning than in how Jay was feeling!"

It was a close match—but Jay won.

When Jay and Bill Cahan had been tennis adversaries for some time, it occurred to Jay that a photograph of doctor and patient playing tennis might be put in *Memorial Cancer News* as an encouragement to other cancer patients.

Dr. Cahan took the idea one giant step further, presenting it to the American Cancer Society. As a result, the two men were scheduled to meet for a tennis game that would be taped and used as a commercial for national television. This commercial, shot over a period of eleven grueling hours, has appeared on national television for the past three years. In addition, a photograph of the tennis match has been published in numerous newspapers and magazines to advertise the Society.

Other media coverage has resulted from the commercial.

In 1981 TSB, Ted Turner's national cable television station in Atlanta, did a special on the American Cancer Society, with one spot featuring a discussion of patient participation by Dr. Cahan and Jay. On another occasion, the two men played tennis for a ten-minute spot on a CBS program.

Jay is presently excited about a project called CAN (Corporate Angel Network) to fly patients to comprehensive cancer centers when necessary. This idea grew out of the observation of Pat Blum, a friend and a recovered mastectomy patient, that many corporate planes left Westchester Airport half empty. Pat, a pilot herself, had seen some planes fly out entirely empty to pick up an executive in another city. She wanted to see companies volunteer their empty seats for cancer patients who might otherwise not go to research centers. Because she was not having much luck implementing this idea, Pat brought it to Jay.

Jay presented the idea to the American Cancer Society, which offered its support. Today the Society does all the preliminary checking of patients who request free flight service. Jay has been primarily concerned with enlisting corporations to donate space in their aircraft, and his success rate has been excellent. Over twenty large corporations are now volunteering their thirty planes. Additionally, Jay's company, Avis, will provide ground transportation wherever possible.

With obvious satisfaction Jay tells about the first patient who used the transportation service, a nineteen-year-old boy who had lost part of a leg to cancer. In December 1981 the program was inaugurated when the boy was flown in a Safe-Flight Instrument Corporation plane from Westchester to Detroit to spend the Christmas holidays with his family.

As impressive as this new concept is—and Jay is confident it will result in a national transportation network for cancer patients—it is his one-to-one volunteer work which he finds most gratifying. Before his illness Jay had been minimally interested in charitable work, although he had been a Boy

Scout leader ("only because my son was in the Scouts") and had worked for the United Fund. Today he devotes a sizable portion of his time to visiting with other cancer patients. As a survivor, he brings hope and inspiration to them.

The staff members at Sloan-Kettering feel that "Jay Weinberg is an absolute wonder. He's come here and visited many patients who are scheduled for similar surgery." As he makes the rounds of a floor, Jay will stroll into a patient's room and begin talking casually. "At first I don't identify myself as someone who's had cancer," he says. "It's a casual approach; I'm a volunteer worker, that's all. So we chat for a while, and then maybe there's a right time to say something about what I went through.

"Often they're shocked, and they say, 'You mean *you* had cancer? But you look so healthy!'

"So I tell them what I went through, and of course they can see how well I've recovered.

"Sometimes when people despair, they'll ask me, 'How can I get up and walk when I feel so rotten?'

"And I tell them, 'You just do it. You just get up and take a step. You've got to believe in yourself and your recovery. Face it—there's no alternative.'"

2

LYNN GRAY

On January 1, 1972, Lynn Gray spent a quiet moment reflecting on her plans for the coming year. She would devote a major portion of her energies to educational reform. Starting a new job as an educational consultant for the Pittsburgh Model Cities Program, she would implement peer teaching programs, where students help teach one another.

Energetic and active, Lynn would continue to fill her life with causes, conduct workshops for teachers, serve on boards dealing with education, manage her household, and spend a good deal of time with her husband, Bob, an insurance broker, and their three children. She would also play as much tennis as possible.

She enjoyed her hectic schedule—always busy and always under pressure to get things done. "I love my life," she thought that day. "Everything I do is important."

During a routine breast self-examination a few days later, Lynn felt a small lump in her right breast and immediately consulted a doctor. However, the doctor could not feel the lump. Unconvinced, Lynn saw a second doctor, who agreed with the first—no lump. Maybe she was imagining it, she thought, and didn't bring up the subject again until she was undergoing a routine annual physical several months later. Again the doctor couldn't locate the lump Lynn was certain she felt, but because of her family history—her mother and two aunts died of cancer—he ordered a mammogram, "to be on the safe side."

"It was there on the mammogram," Lynn says, "the lump nobody thought I had . . . except me. I should have seen another doctor sooner. I should have insisted on a mammogram right away. I'm convinced now that *nobody knows your own body like you do.*"

Lynn was not devastated when the doctor told her she should have a biopsy under a general anesthetic and warned her that if the tumor was malignant, the breast would be removed during the same operation.

"I know lots of women who have had biopsies," she said, "and the tumors have turned out to be benign."

"Your tumor looks malignant," the doctor cautioned her. Nevertheless, Lynn expected to be proved right again.

Lynn entered the hospital under the impression that if the tumor was malignant, at most the breast would be removed. The tumor was malignant, and a mastectomy was performed on the right side. It was several days after the operation when she learned that more than the breast had been removed. She had had a Halstead radical mastectomy. In this operation the breast, underarm tissue, and pectoral muscle are removed. (She would be one of the last women to have this extensive procedure. The important pectoral muscle is no longer removed, because its removal does not decrease the chances of a recurrence of cancer.)

Lynn was angry. "I should have been told, given options. The doctor didn't explain and didn't tell me what he did until therapy to regain the use of my right arm had begun."

In questioning the surgeon, Lynn learned that of the twenty-three lymph nodes he removed, eighteen were found to be malignant. "I was unhappy that I wasn't told what might happen, but I was satisfied that after such extensive surgery there would not be a recurrence." Lynn was relieved to see that the scar on her chest was not as bad as she had feared. "I was expecting to look like a bomb had landed on me," she explains. "I had always heard the words 'mutilating' and 'disfiguring' used to describe a mastectomy. I wish they'd stop using those words—they're very frightening, and I'm sure that the notion of disfigurement prevents many women from getting early diagnosis and early surgery.

"It's really not so terrible," she adds. "You look just like anyone else with your clothes on. To tell the truth, I think a woman who is fifteen pounds overweight is voluntarily disfiguring herself considerably more. I've always been slender, and before the operation I liked my figure. I don't feel any differently now."

During her eight days in Pittsburgh's West Penn Hospital, Lynn was helped by visits from volunteers for Reach to Recovery, an organization which gives support and advice to mastectomy patients. The booklet they left included an exercise program for restoring the usefulness of the affected arm; Lynn followed the exercises religiously, marking her progress with little pencil marks on the wall.

"But what the booklet said about clothing was depressing," she adds. "The idea of having all your clothes made over suggested that you would be very changed. I haven't had to do that at all. I still wear all the same things—tennis clothes, everything. There are very few styles that I can't wear. The booklet also told you to get a bathing suit with a big rubber flower on the shoulder. Ever since I read that, when I see a woman in a bathing suit with a big rubber flower on the shoulder, I think, 'Aha! A mastectomy patient.' I don't have a flower on my bathing suit, and I don't have a problem."

After learning the results of Lynn's surgery, Bob Gray sat down at the telephone, as he had when each of their three children was born, and called everyone close to Lynn. The

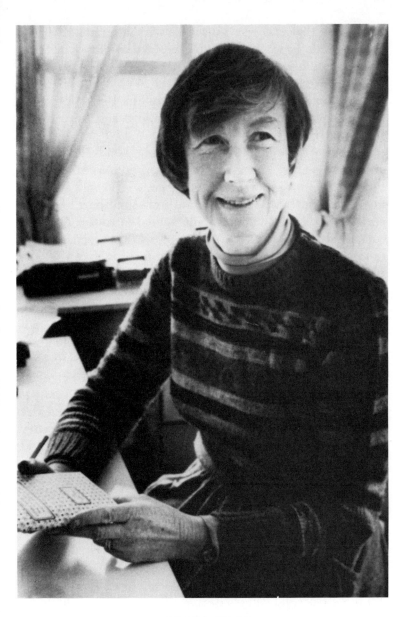

LYNN GRAY

result was that she was showered with attention. "I loved every minute of it. It's a terrible mistake to hide something like this; you need the support of your friends, and you've got to let them know the bad news along with the good news. When cancer became a big part of my life, I couldn't imagine hiding it from my friends. Their love and support has significantly helped my recovery."

When Lynn left the hospital, Bob suggested she consider visiting a cancer clinic. She was surprised. "I thought the surgery did its job, the cancer was gone, and I could go about my life as usual. My ignorance was just astonishing!"

After much consideration Lynn agreed to go to a local oncologist, who prescribed a series of weekly chemotherapy treatments that would take about six months. Lynn is now convinced that such a follow-up with an oncologist is vitally important. "So many patients rely too much on their surgeons after the surgery is complete. I think the follow-up decision should be made by an oncologist—radiation therapy, chemotherapy, or no therapy at all—and that surgeons should automatically send their patients to an oncologist after surgery."

The thank-God-they-got-it-all-out syndrome is a dangerous one, Lynn believes. "I tell other cancer patients that *complacency can kill.* You've got to have a healthy respect for this disease—it is a killer. Once you've had cancer, you had better consider yourself a cancer patient for the rest of your life, and take certain precautions. You need to work to build a high level of wellness, through a healthy life-style, stress management, proper diet and exercise, and avoidance of cancer-causing materials."

Lynn's first chemotherapy treatment was unpleasant. She became nauseated and stayed that way all week. Then the doctor reduced the dosage, and after that she had little nausea and no other side effects.

Long before she had completed the course of chemotherapy, Lynn was back in her regular routine, working and taking care of the house and family. Within five weeks she was playing tennis, enjoying the game as much as ever. She loved the pace and challenge of tennis, and her doctors were amazed at the important muscle development she had achieved through playing.

Shortly after her surgery Lynn (a Sarah Lawrence graduate) decided to get a master's degree in education and enrolled at the University of Pittsburgh. She was involved in her studies, her job, and all her other activities when, in the spring of 1974, she found a lump on her left breast. Immediately she saw a doctor who, after palpating the lump, told her it was benign. Unsatisfied with this diagnosis, Lynn went to her gynecologist; her reaction was the same. But sensing Lynn's worry, she said, "If it will make you feel any better, we can do a biopsy."

Lynn wanted a definitive answer on the lump, but hated the idea of dropping everything to go back in the hospital for the biopsy, which would require a general anesthetic.

"I've been planning on going in for a minor operation on my nose, a deviated septum," Lynn said. "Can we do this during the same hospital stay, so I don't waste any time?" The doctor agreed.

The biopsy was done first, but the nose surgery was canceled because the tumor proved malignant. When Lynn regained consciousness, she learned that a second mastectomy had been performed. The surgery showed further news which was both good and bad: the lymph nodes were not affected. This meant the cancer had not metastasized. But it also meant the tumor was primary, a fresh occurrence of cancer that had nothing to do with the previous lump.

When Lynn entered the hospital for the second operation, she had completed eighteen months of course work for her master's degree. She continued to work on her thesis during her hospitalization. The absorbing, challenging work of the thesis was a great distraction from her physical problems, and kept her involved in the life she had been living.

The surgeon and the oncologist agreed on a course of radiation treatments this time, five a week for five weeks. Lynn drove to the hospital for these treatments, which lasted approximately twenty minutes and had no physical side effects. The emotional effects were another story.

To begin with, she had to wait an hour or more for each treatment. "I felt degraded—like my time was not important. It made me feel like a second-class citizen," she says emphatically. "People there were superficially courteous, but I always felt I was being herded around, or batted from one person to another, like the bird in a badminton game.

"I was unavoidably late for one appointment with the doctor. The nurse asked for an explanation. I felt like I should have a note from my mother! But I just apologized. And then, to punish me, they made me wait another two hours!"

Waiting for radiation treatment was always emotionally upsetting to Lynn. The waiting room often held many patients in advanced stages of cancer, some lying on carts, others unable to sit upright in their wheelchairs. "I was terribly frightened to see patients who were in such bad shape," Lynn says. "It scares me to think about being so debilitated. I think it's bad for the healthier patients to be with the very sick ones. It might be difficult to solve this problem, but one way might be to schedule them at different times of the day."

To keep her spirits up and maintain her sense of dignity, both in treatment and in hospital confinement, Lynn began to surround herself with whatever was individually hers. In her outpatient visits for treatment, she made a point of wearing clothes that expressed her identity; sometimes she came from the tennis court, still in her tennis outfit. To the hospital she brought family photographs and ski and tennis posters for the walls—reminders of good things in her life—and her own print sheets and pillowcases. "It gives some people a start to see the wild-flower prints all over the bed," she says, "but nobody has ever told me not to do it. It helps give me a feeling of identity—I'm a person, not just another case. So does dressing in daytime clothes as much as I can, rather than being in a hospital gown in bed. If I'm dressed and sitting in a chair in my room I don't look like a patient, and I try not to feel like one either."

The radiation treatments were followed by a six-month program of chemotherapy in the form of Alkeran, a pill she took several times a day without any adverse side effects. She was now feeling well and fully active again. Her busy life was interrupted periodically for brain, liver, and bone scans, but she came to expect that she would never have cancer again, and seldom thought about recurrence. For almost three years she remained healthy and symptom-free.

Then, in 1977, she woke up one morning to find nodules an inch in diameter on the surface of her chest. Very frightened, she immediately called the doctor, who scheduled a biopsy. She had no doubt this time that they were malignant—and she was right.

The doctors made it quite clear that the cancer was incurable. They would try to arrest it, of course, and keep her alive and healthy as long as possible.

Radiation treatments were prescribed again. In the meantime, with every day that passed, more nodules appeared, at least two a day, sometimes four. "By the time I saw the doctor at the end of the week," she says, a little pale at the recollection, "I had thirty malignant nodules on my chest. I was absolutely terrified. I knew that I would die soon.

"Following the initial shock, I did a lot of thinking and a lot of praying. It was a difficult process coming to terms with my cancer, and my approaching death."

Lynn has come to the conclusion that most cancer patients, and often their families, once they learn they are in serious trouble, go through the stages of grief usually associated with a death in the family. The first of these is shock. Obviously, the patient who is in shock cannot take an active role in the recovery process, which Lynn believes is essential. The next stage, for many, is denial, either by the patient or the family. "I have never had any problem, nor has my family, with being realistic about my situation," Lynn says. The cancer victim may suffer fear, anger, bewilderment, guilt, depression, a sense of futility, and loss of self-esteem. These emotions and the stress they cause may interfere with the ability of the body's natural immune system to fight and destroy cancer cells.

Ideally, the patient and family will reach a state of acceptance combined with a determination to do everything in their power to make a life with cancer as good a life as possible. Lynn suggests that cancer patients surround themselves with their own therapeutic communities of family and friends. "This means working out any conflicts that may exist," she notes. "Family counseling can sometimes be helpful here.

"My religion has been a great source of strength for me. It gives me a sense of meaning and direction. People all over the country write that they are praying for me, and I can feel the power of their prayers. I pray for them, too."

As Lynn fought through the strong emotions that accompanied this latest malignancy, she began the daily radiation treatments. This time, however, she decided to take them at another hospital. She had become more and more dissatisfied with the autocratic way decisions had been made about her therapy at the first hospital and with the long waits for treatment. She was far happier with the procedures at the new hospital. Most important, after five weeks of daily visits the nodules did go away. In the process Lynn suffered a painful third-degree burn, but she was inexpressibly relieved by the effectiveness of the treatment.

For almost two years Lynn was again symptom-free. Then

the nodules reappeared. More radiation treatments were prescribed, but before long it became clear that Lynn might suffer permanent tissue damage if the treatments were continued. She talked to her doctor about hormone treatment, a promising therapy she had read about for those with breast cancers which are hormone-dependent. Another biopsy was necessary; the results, to Lynn's joy, showed that her cancer was hormone-dependent. This meant that instead of radiation she could be given hormone therapy. The doctor's choice was tamoxifen citrate, and it worked like a charm. Within a few months, the terrifying nodules were gone.

Now Lynn experienced a strange and exciting adjustment. Until the discovery that her cancer was hormone-dependent, she had been resigned to an early death. "Now, suddenly, death was not imminent! So I had to make another adjustment—I had to adjust to living! It sounds strange, but this is a major adjustment, too. I could think in long-range terms, I could plan for the future—I was very excited!" With new confidence Lynn again plunged into her various activities.

Then one morning while on a ski trip with her children she awoke to discover another nodule on her chest. Frightened and downhearted, she called her doctor. "You don't need to jump on the next plane," he told her. "Just stay calm and finish your vacation, and I'll see you when you get back." Lynn decided not to tell the children, but to enjoy this time together. She would inform the whole family when they were back home.

Although Lynn kept this unhappy information from the children for a few days, it had been her policy to tell them the truth about all aspects of her illness. At the time of her first mastectomy David was twelve, Tom was ten, and Laura was nine, too young to be told about cancer, many people would have felt. Lynn strongly disagreed. "It's very important that children are not denied the truth about a serious illness in the family," she says. "You can't deceive them for long. They know something's wrong—they're not stupid. And it's insulting and degrading to them to be left out. When you withhold information, the message they get is, 'You are not responsible enough, not old enough, not smart enough to be told the truth.' It's hard enough on a child to have a parent with cancer, without having to suffer these other psychological problems."

Lynn has been careful to spare her children—and others— the more frightening details of her bouts with cancer. She believes that parents, in talking to their children, must express hope and confidence.

"I recall being told about my mother's condition," she says, shaking her head in disapproval. "The doctor simply said, 'She has cancer and has only six months to live.' You would not want to say that to a child. Instead, you should say something like, 'Mom's got cancer, and it's serious. The doctors are going to do everything possible for her. But we don't know what's in store.'"

No matter how difficult it is for a parent to tell children about cancer, Lynn believes it must be done: "If you don't, their fears will be far worse than the truth. And you can't assume they're not frightened, no matter how cheerful they may seem. You have to give thought to how you can talk with them about it and help them deal with their fears. I always worked hard at communicating with the children. Laurie in particular seemed to have no distress at all about my health. She always seemed happy; she's a euphoric type. But I wondered about it, and one day I asked her, 'Honey, are you scared about me?'

"She immediately said, 'Are you kidding? I'm scared silly!'"

Lynn believes deeply in the parent's responsibility to help children through their own adjustments. In her discussions with and observations of other cancer patients, she has become aware of the many ways children may respond to the news that a parent has cancer. One is through "distancing."

"This is a process in which the child becomes less affectionate and less demonstrative," she explains, "and begins to avoid spending time with the parent. I have known the parent to misunderstand this distancing and be hurt, feeling that the child doesn't care. But I believe it is really an unconscious attempt on the child's part to become more independent—so that when the day comes that the parent is gone, the child can survive and be less devastated by the loss. If you understand this behavior, you can communicate with the child, and explain, 'The closer we are now, the more strength you will have to carry on without me, if you have to.' Children who can express their fears gain the strength and inner security they are going to need to carry on in the event of death."

For Lynn, the thought of her children being without her has been one of the most painful aspects of her illness. "I dearly love my husband, and we have had a wonderful marriage," she says slowly. "I know Bob will go through a tough time when I'm gone, but nothing compared to what the children will go through. I can be replaced as a wife, but as a mother . . . they are not going to replace me. Over the years that I've lived with cancer, I have grieved more for them than for myself. Once I'm gone, I'm out of it—but they're still here, and they have to deal with their loss."

By the time the family returned from their ski trip, there were a few nodules, but this time they were not increasing as quickly as before. The doctor wanted to take a wait-and-see approach, but Lynn was uncomfortable with the situation, and consulted other doctors. She received a wide range of opinions, ranging from additional hormone treatment to extensive chemotherapy. "It's so difficult when you get so many different opinions," she comments. "You don't know what to do. The patient and family always have to make the ultimate decision, but it's hard when there's no consensus among the medical community. And indecision is psychologically more difficult than taking action. But there was such a difference of opinion that I did remain in the wait-and-see posture. The nodules didn't get any worse, but they didn't go away either. They just stayed there, a constant reminder of a dangerous illness."

Lynn continued with her work. She conducted peer-teaching courses for teachers at Penn State University. The time and stress management courses she had been conducting for business and educational institutions led naturally into courses for cancer patients and health care professionals. "Helping others is essential," she says. "It's what keeps people alive." For twenty years she had spent time and energy organizing programs based on people helping other people. She often devoted forty to fifty hours a week as a volunteer or as a professional to such programs. Now she focused on helping cancer patients, and in doing so she felt revitalized. "Being busy and unselfish is very therapeutic," she says.

Her therapy was at a standstill when a friend, who is a physician, told Lynn about a promising new treatment being used in a Philadelphia hospital. Lynn weighed every word as her friend described the use of massive doses of methotrexate (thirty to forty times higher than usual), given intravenously for a period of five days each month.

Lynn was very interested, and soon she and her husband met with the doctor in charge of the program and decided to try it; her reluctance to take five days a month out of her life for treatment was outweighed by the hope the program promised her. The treatment itself was relatively painless. During her five days in the Philadelphia hospital, she was hooked up to an intravenous feeder, receiving first high doses of methotrexate and then Leucovorim calcium injection, a drug to counter its toxic effects. The first day of each month's treatment, Lynn experienced extreme nausea, but the remaining four days were tolerable.

Some of the patients who received the treatment reported positive results and seemed to be in remission. They all had far less nausea than they had experienced with conventional treatment. Lynn was disturbed, however, by the debate over the effectiveness of the treatment for breast cancer, especially when local physicians she talked to expressed doubt. It soon became clear, too, that going to Philadelphia for treatment was more of a problem than she had anticipated. It was impossible to predict whether a bed would be available when Lynn was scheduled. Since she had commitments to lectures and workshops, she needed to know. But her attempts to convince the staff of that were fruitless.

"What's more important, your work or your life?" they would ask.

There was no way of knowing how much good the treatment had done Lynn, but she had lost confidence in it. After five months during which there were no discernible results, she decided to discontinue the program and rely on conventional chemotherapy treatment in Pittsburgh.

For about a year everything went well and Lynn was symptom-free. Then, in 1980, a routine bone scan revealed metastasis to the bones, primarily in the sternum—very disturbing news. But the doctors recommended no treatment for this new cancer; it was not spreading and caused no pain or other symptoms. Lynn was unaffected by it—except for the anxiety of knowing it was there.

Something of a more serious nature showed up on a bone scan a year later—a dark spot in the area of the kidneys. This was very disturbing and very frightening. The nodules on Lynn's chest, like the metastasis to her bones, were stable and did not seem to be life-threatening. "But the kidney news was bad news, and it shook up all of us—Bob, our kids, my friends—all of us," Lynn confides. "All sorts of horrible thoughts went through my mind. I visualized myself on a dialysis machine; I imagined my kidneys failing. Overnight the whole picture changed—from good to bad."

Because it is unusual for breast cancer to metastasize to the kidneys, Lynn's doctor recommended a battery of tests; the results were inconclusive. Then, just before Christmas, there was more bad news. An X ray showed that Lynn's ureters were almost completely blocked, a sign of probable cancer metastasis to that area. Oddly, Lynn experienced no pain or loss of normal function from this, but she was in critical danger; if the ureters are blocked, waste backs up into the kidneys and the overload is progressively more damaging. An exploratory operation was now a necessity.

The physician thought there was no harm in letting Lynn spend Christmas with her family. On January 2, 1982, she was admitted to the hospital, and a few days later the operation took place. The objective was to explore for cancer, remove it if discovered, and free the blocked ureters. "The operation was a failure, but the patient lived," Lynn said later. The cancer was so extensive that the surgeon didn't attempt to remove it, nor was it possible to free the blocked ureters. "I awoke to learn that I was in a heap of trouble—I had inoperable cancer in a vital organ."

But just when her prospects looked worse than ever, her oncologist found a therapy. A biopsy showed that again the metastasis was hormone-dependent; Lynn was put on a different hormone, aminoglutethimide (which has since been withdrawn because of its bad side effects). This treatment works by suppressing the adrenal glands. The hormone is taken along with cortisone, to replace the cortisone the adrenal glands would normally produce. The therapy has been little short of miraculous. The malignant nodules on her chest disappeared, her most recent CAT scan revealed considerably less mass in the kidneys, and she didn't even experience any of the side effects related to aminoglutethimide. Against the odds, the therapy has beaten back the metastasis.

For Lynn, the past ten years have been a roller coaster of dangerous developments, medical successes, and medical failures. This alteration of hope and fear can be maddening, but

Lynn has worked hard to understand the cancer and the emotional problems that accompany it. And she has arrived at a state of calm acceptance. She is able to say matter-of-factly, "This treatment may or may not bring about total remission, but as I understand it, it's likely that the cancer cells will adjust to the new medication within a year or so, and begin to multiply again. I don't think they've come up with a permanent solution, and nobody has promised me one. So I'm simply enjoying every day of good health that I have—and I do feel very good."

Despite the uncertainty of her condition, and the string of frightening recurrences she has faced, Lynn has never asked the classic question, "Why me?" To her, the question is illogical. "One out of every four people will eventually contract some form of cancer. So it's really not so amazing that I'm one of them.

"I can handle this life-threatening situation because my life is so fulfilling. I enjoy each day more than I ever have. I know the joy of loving family and a good marriage. My children are a source of satisfaction and pride—they enjoy me and I enjoy them. I have the support and pleasure of dear friends. I have my work, and my play. There are people who go through life and never have these joys; I've been very lucky, and these satisfactions have made dealing with cancer much easier for me."

In order to perpetuate her work in helping others deal with cancer, Lynn has founded the Lifeline Institute, a nonprofit organization.

"It took me so long to learn what I know about living with cancer," she explains. "I felt I should help others acquire the needed skills more quickly than I did." These skills are discussed in *Living With Cancer*, a basic how-to primer Lynn researched and wrote, and in a cassette she produced, *Mind Over Cancer*, which tells how to cope with stress and harmful emotions and how to use relaxation and imagery techniques to aid recovery. Lynn's lectures and workshops around the country include ones on time management, stress control, taking an active role in the recovery process, and living with cancer. She appears frequently on local and national television shows, and has received thousands of letters asking for her reading and resource lists and brief suggestions for living with cancer. She was recently appointed to the Pennsylvania State Cancer Advisory Board.

Her Lifeline Institute has recently received a grant to expand its programs and create a Cancer Hotline in the Pittsburgh area. The Hotline is based on the innovative and successful telephone service established by Richard Bloch in Kansas City. The service is tied in with an existing crisis hotline, and a troubled cancer victim can receive support, information, and guidance from a trained volunteer who has also experienced cancer. The person who needs help can turn to the volunteer as often as is needed. The Hotline will build a network of people helping people. "Helping others keeps people alive," Lynn says.

She goes on to add, "I want to live long enough to see Lifeline Institute grow and flourish. I want to see millions of people benefit from the booklet and tape, the television shows, the lectures, and the Hotline. That's a long-range goal that keeps me going."

Lynn deeply believes that cancer patients should make a special effort to set goals for themselves. "I've known patients who just *had* to be around long enough to see one of their children marry or graduate from college, or to complete their new house and move in, or to finish writing a book. Many times these people do live to enjoy these events. Then it's important to set new goals for the future, so there is always a good reason to stay alive and healthy."

Lifeline Institute's approach to cancer management begins with helping patients understand the disease, the nature of their own illnesses, and the choices of therapy. Lynn believes patients must participate in decisions as to their therapy, and to do this they must have the facts on hand.

"More patients with cancer discontinue their therapy before the recommended time than patients with other illnesses," she notes. "In one way, this is understandable. Today, many cancers are diagnosed at an early stage, when the patients still feel good; they have cancer, but they're symptom-free. With other illnesses, they go to the doctor feeling terrible, and receive some type of treatment to make them feel better. But with cancer, you usually feel well; then the doctor says, 'You may feel fine, but you have a dangerous illness. We'll give you treatment, and frankly, it's liable to make you feel rotten.' A patient can make decisions on therapy intelligently if he or she really understands cancer and its response to various treatments, as well as the problems to be expected with the therapy. Without treatment you may feel well in the early stages, but you may be throwing away your life.

"Many patients make bad decisions regarding treatment because they are told about the recommended treatment at a time when they cannot respond intelligently to what the physician is saying. They are told immediately after they have been given the diagnosis—which is the correct time, but which is also a point when they are likely to be in the first stage of grief, shock, or in the second emotional stage, denial. Whatever the emotional condition of the patient, I recommend that more than one person be present for the discussion of therapy. Another person will get a different perspective and think of additional questions."

The physician is only one source of information, Lynn points out. Most public libraries contain books on cancer (which may, however, be outdated) and periodicals with up-to-date articles. She recommends talking to nurses, particularly oncological nurse specialists, who often have more time than the physicians and are a source of good information. She also urges patients to get in touch with the National Cancer

Institute's cancer information service. "They provide excellent information on various types of cancer and treatment, and they publish a number of useful pamphlets and booklets." The national toll-free number for this service is (800) 638–6694. The local branch of the American Cancer Society is another recommended source of information, and it provides many services to patients as well. Self-help organizations, such as Make Today Count, can also be very helpful, not only in discussing the disease and emotional reactions, but in evaluating physicians and the various forms of treatment. The Reach to Recovery, Lost Chord, and the Ostomy Association programs have a volunteer who has experienced the same operation call on a patient in the hospital.

"One important effect of learning as much as you can about your illness," Lynn says, "is that it gives you a sense of control over your own body. A real danger of cancer is the feeling of helplessness, and if you simply turn your body over to someone and say, 'Here I am—see what you can do,' you increase this helplessness. When you take an active part in the decision-making process, you gain some control over your illness and your life—and emotionally this is very positive."

Relaxation and stress management are taught on Lifeline's tape, *Mind Over Cancer*. In 1976 Lynn began to learn these skills in a biofeedback clinic at Western Psychiatric Hospital (she notes that her medical insurance covered the cost). The clinic taught Lynn how to reduce the stress in her life, not by changing her life, but by changing her attitude toward the stresses she experienced and by learning to relax. She admits she was a classic "uptight" personality, operating at a dangerously high stress level. She is now able to shrug off little annoyances. "I've always been pretty good with the big things," she comments. "It's the little things that used to upset me, like poor service in a restaurant, or forgetting my briefcase and being forced to waste time going back. Through daily sessions of relaxation and imagery, I've learned to ignore those little irritations and not get so upset. I can handle the stressful aspects of my life very much better."

A time set aside for total relaxation is a daily feature of Lynn's life. She is enthusiastic about imagery techniques to relax her body and mind, and to help activate her body's natural immunity system to fight the cancer cells. She even uses the imagery techniques, which she discusses on her tape, to improve her writing and lecture skills and her tennis. "And you'd be surprised how it's improved my net game! Skiing is also a very mental sport, and imagery has helped me ski faster and with more confidence."

Lynn jogs or bicycles almost every day before breakfast, and when the weather is bad, she runs up and down the stairs in her house fifteen times. "Cancer patients shouldn't perceive themselves as sick people," she says. "Except for the touch of cancer, I *am* a healthy person! Like anyone else, I have to work at maintaining good health." This includes following a nutritional program built around fresh fruits and vegetables, whole grains, fish, and fowl. Lynn avoids sugar, caffeine, refined flour, red meat, junk foods, and deep-fried foods. In her opinion, this diet is one that should simply be followed by anyone who wants optimal health.

Every cancer patient faces difficult emotional adjustments. "You have to be willing to discuss feelings openly and share your problems with others," Lynn says. "It is very important for family and friends to deal with the patient's feelings, by reflecting them and giving the patient a chance to express them freely. I also believe that almost everyone experiencing the gravity of cancer can benefit from counseling of one kind or another. It can be with a psychiatrist or psychologist, a social worker, a minister, or perhaps another cancer patient who is skilled in human relations. I do a great deal of counseling myself.

"Well-meaning friends and family members are not always helpful when it comes to dealing with painful feelings. A cancer patient may say, for instance, 'I'm really frightened. I don't think I'm going to live to see my son's graduation.' A friend or relative might respond, 'Oh, you'll outlive all of us.' Well, that is *not* a productive thing to say. It is a total denial of the feelings the patient needs to express. Instead, the other person should acknowledge and sympathize with the patient's feelings and say something like, 'It's good that you're upset now about your future. . . . You should be upset. . . . But don't forget you have a future. . . .'

"If a person responds to a patient's emotional statements with a remark that denies the emotion, the cancer patient can reply, 'What you just said is not helpful to me at all. Let's deal with what's worrying me.'

"Another very unhelpful remark people will make is, 'Oh well, we've all got to die sometime.' When you have cancer, that is hardly what you need to hear. After all, some of us are more mortal than others!"

For Lynn, communication skills, like self-education and decision making, are ways cancer patients can control their lives instead of feeling trapped helplessly by illness. "Your cancer may not go away," she says, "but you may live a lot longer and be in much better condition by taking command of your own body and life. And your days will surely be happier for you and those you care about."

The belief that cancer patients should make their own decisions is one Lynn extends to every facet of cancer treatment. She believes there may come a time when an informed patient feels that treatment is more painful than productive. The decision to discontinue a treatment which has very debilitating side effects is one she thinks is well within the patient's rights. "If there is obviously not much time left, and discontinuing treatment will improve the quality of that time, who's to say this is not the right decision?"

For Lynn Gray, a ten-year survivor, the quality of life has never been better. She sums up, "I believe there's a high-level wellness which transcends all illness—a wellness of the spirit that is more important than wellness of the body. In this respect, it's been said that Hubert Humphrey died a well man. I believe that's true. And I feel I have attained that wellness of the spirit and serenity—even what I might call a feeling of joy. If the spirit is healthy, the body cannot be defeated."

3

SHAINDY FENTON

A recent article in *Harper's Bazaar* titled "Five Winning Women from Texas" included Lady Bird Johnson—and Shaindy Fenton. Shaindy who?

Shaindy herself admits, "I am not famous like a movie star is famous. But in the art world I am very famous. There is no one who collects or sells contemporary art who doesn't know my name. I'm not bragging; it's a simple fact." In the art world, Shaindy is a superstar. Andy Warhol has twice painted her portrait. Isamu Noguchi, the famous Japanese-American artist, has dedicated sculpture to her. Roy Lichtenstein has come to visit her hospital bed. She has bought art from the Rockefellers. And Stanley Marcus, of Neiman-Marcus department stores, says of Shaindy, "She has an incomparable knowledge of the art market."

Shaindy is also a striking beauty, dark-haired, fair-skinned, and resembles an artist's model more than a shrewd, aggressive art dealer. She wears a Roberto Cavalli suede dress at the time of this interview, and the hand-painted gold and turquoise flowers of the design set off her long hair and dark eyes. She also wears original art, a necklace made by Man Ray, the famous surrealist, and a gold bracelet and rings. If all this sounds expensive, it is. "I spend between $30,000 and $40,000 a year on clothes," she says matter-of-factly. But she can afford to. In 1981, she sold over $10 million worth of art to her more than one hundred clients.

All this Shaindy does out of her home in Fort Worth, Texas—not exactly the art capital of the world. Since there's a limited market for Frank Stellas, Jean Dubuffets, Roy Lichtensteins, Jasper Johnses, and Andy Warhols in Fort Worth, most of Shaindy's clients are out of town. To meet with them, and to acquire paintings, she travels all over the United States. When she isn't traveling, her husband, Bob, and their teenage son, Keith, know where to find her: sitting in bed, surrounded by art books and brochures, and talking long-distance—which she usually does for seven or eight hours a day.

Since only a handful of galleries in the world sell $10 million worth of art a year, it would be natural to assume that Shaindy is one of those firecracker entrepreneurs with a boundless supply of energy, enthusiasm, and good health. Her energy and enthusiasm are amazing, but her health is far from good. She suffers from a rare hereditary disease, von Hippel-Lindau, which claimed the lives of her father, paternal grandmother, and aunt. This unpredictable disease may cause tumors to develop in the eyes, kidney, pancreas, adrenal glands, lungs, and brain. The eye and brain tumors sometimes prove to be benign, but tumors in the other areas are usually malignant. Von Hippel-Lindau is complicated and rare, and leads to a different pattern of symptoms in each patient. For these reasons, it is difficult to diagnose. Victims of von Hippel-Lindau may suffer from a host of problems with no clear, central cause.

Shaindy's troubles began when she was twenty-two years old and pregnant. She and Bob were living in Philadelphia, where he was interning at Bryn Mawr Hospital in preparation for a career as an allergist. Shaindy became concerned about the continuing loss of her hair, and went to Temple University's Skin Cancer Hospital to consult a renowned dermatologist. Her family's history of von Hippel-Lindau was not yet known. Because her parents had divorced when she was a child, she was not aware that her father's sister had died of cancer due to the disease; her father had not yet contracted it. After a battery of tests, the dermatologist was still at a loss as to why her follicles were forming tiny knobs and why the hair was breaking off at these points.

Finally the doctor said, "I've done everything I know how to and I still don't know what's the matter with you. Why don't you go to an internist?"

Immediately, Bob set up an appointment with an internist at Bryn Mawr Hospital. But this visit, too, was unproductive, except that the internist detected "something funny" when he examined Shaindy's eyes. He sent her on to an ophthalmologist.

When Bob got home that evening, and Shaindy told him what the internist had said, Bob examined her eyes himself. Finally he sat back and said, "I see an angioma."

"What is *that?*"

"A tumor, made up of blood vessels or lymph vessels. It could be nothing serious. But you do have to see an ophthalmologist right away."

The eye specialist agreed with Bob's observation, but said he was not the best person to treat the tumor in Saindy's right eye. "No one in Philadelphia is really qualified in this area," he said. "I want you to see a specialist in New York who's been working on developing the argon laser."

The treatment was successful, but as soon as the laser eradicated one tumor, another one appeared.

"I was pregnant," Shaindy says, "and getting more and more pregnant, and still more and more tumors kept coming. No sooner did they knock one out than another one would appear." Shaindy was no complainer, but the treatments

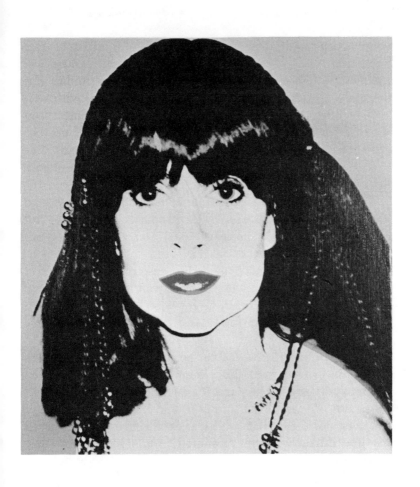

SHAINDY FENTON

(photograph of the oil painting by Andy Warhol)

were not pleasant; the photocoagulation, for instance, was done under local anesthetic administered through a needle in the eye. But more important, the tumors were so prolific that despite everything, Shaindy lost her vision in her right eye.

"The doctors warned me I would probably lose some of my sight, so I was prepared for that. What bothered me was that after my son was born, I started to get tumors on the other eye. *That* scared me to death." These tumors, however, did not affect the optic nerve.

The ophthalmologist knew immediately that Shaindy had von Hippel-Lindau disease. "Most people don't have the full course of the disease," he explained. "You will probably just get it in the eyes and then be fine."

Shaindy nevertheless developed a sense of fatality. "I read in a book that everyone who contracts von Hippel at an early age dies from it before reaching forty. So I decided, okay, I'm going to die before I'm forty. And that totally changed my life.

"Maybe it wasn't reasonable, because in some people the disease never progresses. But I knew that other people get the whole works, everything, and it's awful, and I just knew that I'd be one of them. I felt sure of it, and I accepted it. I didn't roll over and die. What I did was decide that for the rest of my life, I'd do whatever I wanted. And I have. Ever since then, I've done just what I wanted to do."

For the next several years, Shaindy's health remained stable, and the recurring tumors on her left eye finally disappeared. She and Bob moved to Fort Worth, where he opened a practice, specializing in the treatment of allergies.

As Bob's practice grew and the young couple began to buy art for their house, Shaindy's interest and taste became apparent. Before long she ran across a New York dealer in art prints who would sell to her at wholesale prices. That gave her an idea; she could be his Texas representative. The dealer was skeptical. "Your husband's a doctor. He's not going to want you to be a salesperson."

"You don't know Bob," Shaindy said confidently. "He never stops me from doing anything. He always encourages me to be everything I want."

This proved to be true, and soon Shaindy was selling inexpensive prints in the Fort Worth–Dallas area, earning 10 percent commissions. "Then one day, on Bob's afternoon off, I spent the whole day waiting in a client's reception area, and all he bought was one $25.00 print! For $2.50 I killed an entire day, when I could have been with Bob. That's when he said to me, 'Shaindy, if you're going to be in business, make money at it—or forget it!' And I realized he was right."

With his encouragement, Shaindy placed some small ads in medical journals Bob received, and began dealing in prints by well-known artists, such as Matisse, Picasso, and Miró. The mail-order and telephone business was supplemented by sales to people she and Bob had met during his internship and military service. Shaindy's interest in art became a passion; she read everything she could find on contemporary art. Their bedroom, her headquarters, became a virtual art library, with books stacked and shelved everywhere.

Without the academic credentials many dealers point to, Shaindy became a respected dealer before she was out of her twenties, "just by living, eating, and breathing art." She visited galleries around the world, and talked on the phone to experts she couldn't visit in person. Before long she was capable of giving a client, from memory, all relevant information about any important piece of contemporary art, including its sales history over the past ten years. Soon this led to meeting the "right" people, such as the director of the Fort Worth Art Museum; he took her under his wing and introduced her to his contacts, and they in turn introduced her to theirs. Eventually Shaindy Fenton was so well known that clients came to her to introduce themselves. After she helped put together some of the best art collections in America there was no doubt: she had arrived.

In the eighteen years since she learned about von Hippel-Lindau, Shaindy has kept her vow to *live*. If she seems to live fast and hard, no wonder. "I had a timetable that would be expired by age forty," she says. "I had a lot to do in a shorter period of time than most people."

Shaindy's success has taken place against a backdrop of pain and uncertainty, however, for the disease has progressed intermittently during the course of her high-flying life. In 1971, six years after the disappearance of her eye tumors, doctors discovered tumors in her Fallopian tubes which were benign but nevertheless necessitated a hysterectomy. Later developments would show that these tumors were also related to von Hippel-Lindau, but at the time the doctors didn't make that connection. "The tumors on my Fallopian tubes were different from the usual tumor," Shaindy says. "So different that they sent the biopsy slides to doctors all over the country to try to find out what they were. But nobody knew."

Since the tumors had not been malignant, Shaindy refused to be worried by them. In no time she was back on her feet and deeply involved in her business. But suddenly she found herself without the energy to keep up her usual pace.

"I was very tired, just dragging around, having a hard time doing anything. Finally I decided it was my metabolism, and I asked Bob to check it. When he did, he thought I might be diabetic, so he sent me to my internist. Well, it was severe diabetes, and it was caused by more tumors—this time on my pancreas."

The pancreatic tumors had destroyed the ability of Shaindy's pancreas to produce insulin; the internist started her on insulin injections and a diet with no sugar, alcohol, or caffeine. She followed the regimen, willing to do anything that would restore her energy and sense of well-being.

Then one day, sitting next to Bob on a plane going from Florida to Fort Worth, Shaindy felt distinct difficulty in breathing. Bob had never seen anything like it and didn't know what to do; soon the condition eased up a little. The next morning, however, she was still feeling odd and unwell, so Bob took her to the doctor. The verdict was flu. Since it was severe, the doctor asked Shaindy if she wanted to go into the hospital.

"I said no," she recounts with a shrug. "I mean, who wants to go to the hospital?" But while Bob went to get the car, Shaindy grew so weak that she sat down on the pavement in front of the doctor's office. Bob had to pick her up and put her in the car. She argued that once home, she would feel better. Instead she felt worse. Finally Bob put her in the car and took her to a hospital emergency room.

There, Shaindy passed out. The doctors diagnosed diabetic coma, and gave her insulin. The results were amazing. "I felt like I returned from the dead. I just zipped back again."

But of course the problem was not entirely solved. Because Shaindy's adrenal glands were also tumorous now, they were producing a substance that triggered more diabetic comas. She says, "Every so often my breathing would stop and I'd pass out. It was very frightening."

Shaindy left the hospital with the diabetes largely under control. But her doctors did not connect her variety of tumors with von Hippel-Lindau disease. The connection was not made until two years later, in 1979, when shooting pains in her left leg were found to be caused by yet another nonmalignant tumor, this time on a nerve. The tumor was removed. Just two months later, however, other, more mysterious symptoms appeared.

"I was talking on the telephone," Shaindy recalls, "when I had such an awful pain in my side, it took my breath away. Bob had me examined again, and they gave me all kinds of X rays, and then told me nothing was wrong. 'But feel this lump on my stomach,' I'd say. They'd feel it and say, 'It's nothing.'"

But it was something. When Shaindy went in for an insurance physical, having applied to take out a large life policy, the first thing the doctor said was, "There's a lump in your stomach. You'll have to have a CAT scan."

Shaindy told him, "I've been X-rayed four times already, and four times they told me it was nothing."

"No CAT scan, no insurance," he said.

The CAT scan showed a tumor in Shaindy's stomach, and revealed the tumors on her adrenal glands. Needless to say, the insurance company did not issue the new policy. But the examination had pinpointed problems that had evaded the doctors up till then. As a result of that exam, Shaindy again underwent surgery, in which several malignant tumors were removed, along with her left kidney and her adrenal glands.

Equally important, the doctors finally saw the pattern of her disease. They were aided by the autopsy report on Shaindy's father, and they also got the report on her aunt. Both had died of cancer, directly related to von Hippel-Lindau. "Finally the doctors put the whole thing together and decided all my previous tumors were related, and caused by von Hippel-Lindau."

Shaindy understands why the doctors found the cause so difficult to pinpoint. Von Hippel-Lindau is extremely rare and varies from patient to patient. The diagnosis would have been easier with a fuller family medical history. Shaindy had been sure for fourteen years now that she would die of von Hippel, ever since her eye tumors were diagnosed. But it had taken all this time for the doctors to piece together the varying symptoms of her specific disease. When they did, they told Shaindy she was one of the less fortunate victims of this rare disease—she would have the full course. At age thirty-six, she had already had tumors in both eyes, her Fallopian tubes, her pancreas, her adrenal glands, her kidney, her leg, and her stomach.

Then, in December 1980, a chest X ray revealed several tumors in her lung. The doctors felt the best course of action was simply to watch the tumors for a month and see if they changed.

Meanwhile, Bob decided that the best place to go for treatment of von Hippel-Lindau was Philadelphia. After Christmas he and Shaindy flew there, and the doctors took a biopsy of her lung. "Then they looked all the way from the top of my back to the bottom, and found, I don't know, twenty or thirty tumors on my lungs. I don't remember how many, but what difference does it make? There were too many to remove; it would have killed me. They just closed me up."

The exploratory surgery was followed by sophisticated scans to determine if there was any other cancer in Shaindy's body. The biopsy had revealed that the tumors in her lung were malignant, and of a very rare kind—adrenal gland cancer which had metastasized. "It never does that," Shaindy says, "well, almost never—and I have to be the one."

The scans revealed that the cancer which almost never spreads had also spread to Shaindy's remaining kidney, which showed new tumors. The doctor took Bob aside and told him, "There's nothing we can do. Your wife probably has about six months to live."

Shaken, Bob wondered how much to tell Shaindy just then. He had stepped out of the room for a moment when another doctor came in.

"We found all these kidney tumors," he told Shaindy bluntly.

She asked, "What are you going to do?"

"That's just it," he replied, shaking his head. "There's nothing we can do."

Shaindy was frightened. As she sat on her bed she thought,

"When I was twenty-two I knew I'd die before I was forty. Still, it's two different things to read about that at age twenty-two and to hear the sentence pronounced at age thirty-seven."

Bob denied the prognosis. For days, he sat at his desk making one phone call after another, until he got a consensus on who seemed to be the greatest expert on von Hippel-Lindau—Dr. Carl Engleman, in Philadelphia.

"Can you imagine?" Shaindy asks. "Bob called all over the world, and we end up back in Philadelphia again."

She was admitted to the hospital there as Dr. Engleman's patient for two weeks, during which time he ran a battery of tests. The conclusion: The lung tumors were not necessarily killers. "They're very unpredictable," he told Shaindy. "Sometimes they kill you, sometimes they don't. I once had a little girl who had them, and they just disappeared."

This prognosis cheered Shaindy up immeasurably. At the same time, she had to adjust to the frightening possibility that the tumors on her kidney could not be removed without the entire kidney being removed as well.

"That *really* got me," Shaindy says. "That was my only kidney—I'd have to be on dialysis. I had good reason to be scared, and no one could reassure me."

Fortunately, the surgeons were able to remove six tumors from her kidney without taking the kidney itself. After a brief stay in the hospital, Shaindy convinced the doctor to let her convalesce at her brother's home in Philadelphia for a week. Then she was able to go back to Fort Worth.

She was hardly home when more trouble began. Unable to keep anything on her stomach, Shaindy vomited for two days until Bob finally overrode her desire to stay at home, and took her to the hospital. There, extensive tests revealed difficulties stemming from her operations. Painful adhesions had formed. Once again, she would have to have surgery.

"I'm just not going to do it," she said. "That's all there is to it. I'm sick of being operated on!"

"It's nothing much, " she was assured. "This operation will be like having your appendix removed, no worse."

Shaindy remembers that conversation well. Since her appendectomy had been easy, she finally agreed to go through with the "nothing much" operation. "And it was without question absolutely the worst operation I ever had!" she says. "For whatever reason, they had to do the whole thing twice. Afterwards I was in so much pain it hurt just to breathe!"

Shaindy knew she would have to do something to distract herself from the pain. So two weeks after the surgery she flew to St. Louis to visit a client. "That was the first time I was laid up for more than a week after an operation. But going to St. Louis was a victory for me. Forget the business I did there, just getting there was a victory. The pain slowed me up some, but it didn't kill me."

When she returned, however, Shaindy was confronted with yet another problem related to her disease. While she could now breathe with some comfort, she began having pain in her legs. "It was like someone was throwing hot oil on me, except that it was inside, not on the skin. It was excruciating. I was in bad, bad shape. And for months they couldn't find out what it was, and meanwhile I couldn't walk, I couldn't sleep, I couldn't eat. I couldn't do anything. It was awful!"

Driven to distraction by pain, Shaindy decided she could sleep if only she had the right mattress. "That was when I started throwing out beds. I was sure the right bed would help, so I started changing beds, buying one after another. When you don't sleep for weeks and weeks, you get kind of crazy. Finally I realized a new bed wasn't the solution at all."

In their search for solutions, the Fentons turned to neurologists, acupuncturists, and hypnotists. Nothing worked. The problem turned out to be diabetic neuropathy, and the pain continued, no matter what was prescribed for it.

During the months when she was plagued with these shooting pains, Shaindy was in and out of the hospital several

times, receiving dozens of tests. She lost so much weight that
friends were horrified to see her. Previously she had resolved
to go to the Chicago and New York Art Fairs, two of the most
important art fairs in the country. And she did go, even
though the pain was so severe she was unable to keep from
crying on the plane all the way home from the New York
show. When Bob met her at the airport, he took her straight
to the local hospital, where she was given Nubain. This painkiller eased her somewhat, but the only solution to the pains
in her legs turned out to be time; over the months they grew
less severe and finally disappeared.

By now it had been a year since the kidney operation, and
Shaindy had been putting off the necessary kidney test for six
months, because her allergy to the dye injected for the test
caused her to shake uncontrollably. She was convinced to go
back to Philadelphia, however, by the doctor's request to test
her son for von Hippel-Lindau at the same time.

"The news was great! It was all good! My son did not have
von Hippel-Lindau; he looked fine. And my kidney had gone
back to its healthy form; the cuts from the surgery had
healed, and the kidney had actually grown larger. I went
home on a cloud."

The plane had hardly touched down before Shaindy was
once again happily ensconced on her bed, books and papers
spread around her and the telephone in her hand. The doctors had told her not to come back for two years. She was
well.

A few days later, when the Fentons were still getting used
to the good news, Shaindy began vomiting again. The doctor
diagnosed the problem as flu, and had Shaindy admitted to
the hospital. She was no better after three days, and when
Bob heard that Shaindy's vision was almost gone, he became
alarmed. He rushed over and convinced a neurologist to do
an immediate brain scan.

One hour later, Shaindy was once again operated on—this time for the most serious problem of all, a brain tumor. The swelling in her brain was so bad that the tumor could not be immediately removed. Instead, the surgeon had to insert a shunt into Shaindy's brain to relieve the pressure. She awoke three days later to learn that the tumor was not malignant, but had not yet been removed; she would have to stay in the hospital for a week until the shunt relieved the swelling enough for the operation to take place.

Shaindy had been in extreme danger with the tumor; "I was told that my brain would have exploded if they hadn't put the shunt in when they did." The forthcoming operation was also risky. Shaindy had endured much, but she was reaching her limit. "I was so disgusted and upset I didn't open my mouth for the entire week. And I usually talk all the time. Even when my brother came from Philadelphia, I wouldn't talk to him."

But most of all, Shaindy was frightened. "I wasn't afraid of dying, I was afraid they would do something awful to me and I *wouldn't* die. And would be . . . incapacitated in some way." Her dark eyes momentarily shadow. "Being incapacitated, that would be worse to me than dying. I'd rather be dead."

For the only time in all her hospitalizations, Shaindy lay in her hospital bed, inactive. The Rolodex with the names of clients and dealers which she always took with her sat unused. She talked to no one.

The surgery, when it finally took place, was a tremendous relief to all concerned. The tumor was removed, and everything looked fine, although, as the doctor told Shaindy, her husband, and her cousin, she would not be able to walk for about six months. "You'll need to make arrangements for physical therapy," he said.

"Okay," Bob replied. "But she's not going to like this."

Shaindy didn't like it. While the three of them stood discussing her inability to walk, she jumped out of bed and walked across the room toward them.

"You should have seen their expressions!" she says gleefully. "They almost fainted!" She admits that she didn't exactly walk a straight line, and still can't. "So what? Who needs to walk a straight line?"

Shaindy's reaction to the upcoming ordeal of brain surgery was unusual—for her. Remembering it, she says with a puzzled frown, "That's the only time I ever got like that. I didn't work *all week*. Other times, I just kept on going, even from my hospital bed. I remember one time, I forget which operation it was, when they came for me I was talking on the phone, in the middle of this deal. I told them, 'I'm not going till I finish this deal.' And I didn't. I finished what I was doing, and *then* I went for surgery."

While Shaindy's devotion to her business may exasperate hospital personnel, it is one of the things that have kept her alive. "If I didn't have my business, I don't think I'd want to live. Oh, maybe I'd find something else to put my energy into, but if I didn't have *something* like this, I don't think I'd be alive today."

Bob agrees. "Except for the night hours, when we turn off the phone, it rings every five minutes. She might be lying down, not feeling good, but she'll answer a call and just light up. It keeps her moving."

Shaindy keeps the business moving, too, something she has been able to do because much of her work is done on the telephone. Through her most severe pain and illness, with the single exception of the week before the brain surgery, Shaindy has studied, talked, put together deals, and built one of the most significant businesses of its kind in the country. In 1981, one of her worst years in terms of health, she reached a sales volume higher than $10 million—her best year ever.

"But it's Bob who really keeps me alive," she says, "not the business. For one thing, because he's a doctor he knows how to handle problems. And he's very persistent. He'll call people all over the world to get the best medical help for me. He made up his mind to find out everything about this disease, and that's what he's done."

Even Bob has not been able to protect Shaindy from her disease, although he has cushioned the worst of it for her. With his help, her spirits have usually remained high—but not always. Once, a well-meaning relative had Shaindy talk on the phone to a woman in Philadelphia who was also hospitalized with von Hippel-Lindau. "This woman was having trouble with her *second* kidney," Shaindy says, "she was just over forty, and she was blind, *and* her husband had left her. It was so depressing. On top of all that, her nineteen-year-old son had a brain tumor. I'm usually a very positive person, and I feel I can help people, but what could I say to this woman? I said we all put up with whatever we have to, and learn to live with it. But when it's your kid, that's tough."

Shaindy realizes how tough it's been for her son; he's had to live with all her problems and also the threat of getting von Hippel-Lindau himself. "Keith's had some hard times. When I had that terrible leg pain, he could hear me groaning at night in my sleep. I do feel guilty about that. . . . But we've talked and talked to him about this, kept him filled in, and he's the most well-adjusted child you'll ever see."

Shaindy tried to raise Keith the way her mother raised her. "She always told me I was the best, the prettiest, the most wonderful person in the world. And it's like the Montessori system teaches, 'What you think of me, I will think of me, and what I think of me, I will be.' She made me think I was wonderful, and if you think that way, other people will see you that way, too. So I grew up believing I could do anything I wanted to. And I do most everything I set out to do. I know that sounds like bragging, but it's true.

"Besides, when you're twenty-two years old and you read

that you're going to have all these terrible things happen to you, and you're going to die before you're forty—it changes everything. You take stock of your life. How are you going to deal with this?

"My reaction was to live my life on fast time. And it's been a good life, in fact a super life. I have a great family and incredible, wonderful friends, and my clients are like family to me. So I've been very blessed."

With a look of satisfaction, Shaindy concludes, "I've had a very good time. If I were to die tomorrow, life doesn't owe me a nickel."

4

JACOB SNYDER

Jack Snyder was in Mexico when he first noticed minor pains in his chest. This in itself did not alarm him. The raspiness in his voice did not seem very serious either, but the blood he was coughing up worried him.

While he knew these symptoms demanded a doctor's attention, Jack did not feel unduly anxious about them. His work just then, in late 1964, demanded all his attention. Jack was an executive for a publicly owned Israeli real estate development company. Traveling with him and meeting with groups of potential investors was Israel's great military hero, Moshe Dayan.

Disturbed about the blood in his sputum, Jack took time from his meetings to consult a doctor in Mexico City. The diagnosis was "a cold," and the doctor gave Jack medication to relieve the symptoms. The medicine didn't help, but Jack continued traveling with the group from Mexico to Venezuela. By the time he returned to his home in New York, he was weak and quite worried about the blood he was still coughing up. He immediately went to see his doctor.

The physician found no explanation, and referred Jack to another doctor. Eventually cancer was suspected, and Jack was sent to Dr. William Cahan, who suggested an overnight examination, including a bronchoscopy, at Manhattan Eye and Ear.

The following morning Jack and his wife, Faigal, learned what the tests had revealed. Jack had lung cancer.

Not once had Jack seriously considered that he might have cancer. Yet now he simply accepted the diagnosis thoughtfully. "I know that may seem strange," he says. "Many people are shaken to the roots by such news, but I didn't feel as if I had been sentenced to death. I didn't have that sense of imminent doom. I simply said to Dr. Cahan, 'Well, where do we go from here?' "

Although Dr. Cahan may have been surprised by Jack's calm, Faigal knew that, for Jack, it was a typical reaction. Since his graduation from law school in 1942, Jack had been deeply involved in administrative work in one capacity or another (although never as a lawyer, despite the fact that he is a member of the bar). He confronted problems and difficulties daily. It was not his style to brood or get hysterical. Instead, his reaction to adversity—even cancer—was, "Well, what do we do now? Where do we go from here?"

Jack never asked the question, "Why me?" He reminded himself that "the universe is random; the cosmos doesn't play favorites." This attitude, Jack says, "is perhaps both my greatest virtue and my greatest fault. It means I tend to suppress my emotional experiences, to get right down to cases."

Getting down to cases now meant that Jack saw the cancer as an adversary, like any other, and immediately took an adversary position to combat it. "I realized I must marshal my forces," he says, "and work at defeating this disease. I felt I could not rely on any outside, supernatural force to help me. I was in a life-threatening circumstance, and I felt that a man in danger must rely mainly on his own physical and spiritual resources. I was determined to battle this with dignity and courage."

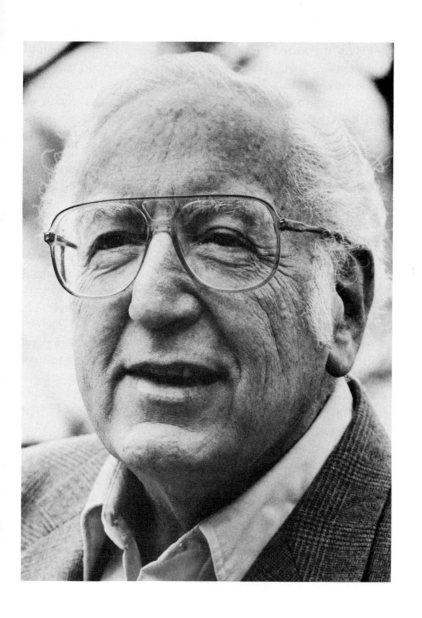

JACOB SNYDER

Faigal supported Jack by concealing her tears and anxiety. The couple, married over twenty years, understood each other's needs. "It's not that we don't have feelings like the next guy," Jack says. "But I wasn't ready to be mourned for. If we had believed there were no alternatives to death, we might have acted very differently.

"I was only forty-seven at that time," he says, "and I had never thought much about dying. Nowadays, naturally, I think a great deal about dying, particularly the philosophic implications of death. But then I just wanted to get on with the business at hand, and find out what I had to do to get well again."

Dr. Cahan's recommendation was radical surgery at Memorial Sloan-Kettering Cancer Center, where he was and is an attending surgeon in the Thoracic Service. The surgery was to be preceded by ten days of radiation treatment "to take the heat off the cancer." Jack appreciated the doctor's direct approach and he trusted Dr. Cahan implicitly. Faigal, a dietitian, had numerous friends in the medical profession; she had talked to them and learned that Cahan's reputation was excellent and that Memorial was considered one of the best cancer research hospitals in the country. Jack felt he could not be in better hands. Without a second opinion, he accepted the diagnosis and treatment plan.

Knowing that he would be convalescent for some time after the surgery, Jack went to the office daily during the preoperative period of radiation treatments. He caught up on paperwork and delegated areas of responsibility to other people, as he might before a prolonged business trip. He knew his staff was competent to handle problems in his absence. When he left the office on the last day, it was with a clear mind and every expectation of returning.

On February 17, 1965, the day before his forty-eighth birthday, Jack underwent surgery. While his attitude was not blithe, he was far less concerned than he would have been if he had known that in the long run he was not expected to survive. "Nobody told me that, and as far as I'm concerned, that's fine—I believe the doctor should be straightforward, but there's nothing to be gained by actually stating odds when they are so bad."

The surgery was extensive. Not only was the major lobe of Jack's right lung removed, but the intercostal tissue (tissue between the ribs) had to be excised because the cancer had spread beyond the lung. This meant that the operation included rebuilding Jack's rib structure with a plastic substitute.

The aftermath of the surgery was extremely painful. The constant pain sharpened with every breath he took. The worst part was that he had to cough deeply several times a day to keep his lungs clear of phlegm. "That was one of the most painful things I've ever experienced," he says. "It was a terrible struggle to actually make myself cough and bring that agony on."

Jack was inquisitive about procedures, and Dr. Cahan and the staff were willing to answer his questions at any time, in as much detail as he wanted. Jack stresses that every patient should ask questions about everything. "Knowing why this and why that had a very positive effect on me," he says. "It gave me a sense of confidence. And it also made it easy for me to be fully cooperative." When Jack asked that his dosage of painkiller be increased, he was told that the only effective pain reliever was also addictive; there was good reason not to escalate his dosage. "Once I knew that," he says, "I had the courage to hold back. But if I had simply been told, 'You can't have it,' without any reason why, I would have been resentful. I was able to endure because I could see that it made sense."

Jack's understanding of the medical decisions motivated him to work toward full recovery. And he believes that his participation was very important. "Take just one thing, like the postsurgical coughing. If I had felt it was all hopeless, I couldn't have endured the pain. I put oomph into the coughing because I understood that this would help me, and because I *believed* I was going to get well. This positive feeling about the future may be a small, subtle difference, but it is what motivates me to tackle those difficult obstacles.

"Positive thinking and hope are vital ingredients in recovery," he adds, "but anyone who ignores medical science and attempts to conquer this disease with thought alone is off base, in my opinion. I don't like illusions, and I believe it's wrong for people to live with false hopes and false expectations.

"That doesn't mean I'm a cynic—far from it. I know that a negative attitude can damage your health. Negative, fearful thoughts are stressful, and stress creates symptoms, even in an otherwise healthy body. So you've got to have a positive approach—there's really no choice."

Jack adds, "Even the most positive cancer patient is bound to have periods of depression. It's ridiculous to think this is all one sweet musical comedy you play out in three acts, and everybody goes away laughing. Don't think there aren't going to be bad days, because there most certainly will be. Although I did not experience severe depression, I had my down days. My family and friends played a major role in lifting me out of them. Little things—a letter, a phone call, somebody dropping by—there's nothing like laughing with friends to lift your spirits.

"Maybe the best way to combat depression is to get on with living. It's easy to say, 'I have this illness, I'm sick, I can't stand up, I can't even go to the toilet alone.' When you carry on that way, you make your own disability. It's bad enough to have an actual disability to cope with; you don't want to compound it by imposing another one on top of it."

For Jack, the modern procedure of quickly getting surgical patients on their feet makes sense. "Nowadays many patients are up and walking the day after surgery," he comments. "I understand this aids healing, but it's also good for your spirit. Instead of lying there helplessly, feeling like a victim, you're on the road to living like a normal human being again."

For nearly two months after his discharge, Jack convalesced at home. At first his right arm was not fully useful, and he continued to experience pain and a general lack of energy. Dr. Cahan put no restrictions on his activities, and predicted that the strength in Jack's arm would return without physical therapy. Slowly it did. Broadening his activity a little each day, and resting a great deal, Jack regained his energy. His two sons and daughter, then teenagers, joined with his wife in reinforcing Jack's progress. Faigal, who was told from the beginning that the odds were against Jack's long-term survival, never showed that in her words or her actions. "Needless to say," he says, "her strength reinforced mine. I feel sorry for the poor guy whose wife is upset and always on the verge of tears. I don't see how you can be full of fight if you're sapping your energy in trying to console someone else."

Jack also had a very special means of support—a group of lifelong friends. "We've been as close as brothers for the past forty-five years or so," he said. "Many, many years ago when we were young men back in Philadelphia, we decided to constitute ourselves transcendental friends, meaning that in the future we would preserve the same high degree of intimacy we felt then, and that it would exist all of our lives.

"And that happened. We felt and still feel a beautiful bond of friendship with one another—something closer, I believe, than most brothers ever share. For all these years our beautiful relationship has persisted. My transcendental friends. We live in different cities now, and two or three years may elapse without our making contact, yet when I pick up the phone and say hello to one of them, it's as if we've been in touch constantly. So of course I heard from each of them during my convalescence, and that was the most wonderful medicine possible."

Jack believes the love of family and friends touches something deeply related to recovery. "Call it a person's spirit, his life force—perhaps it's merely his metabolism. Something important is fed by love and companionship. Lonely people must have a more difficult time recovering from illness. I think people can die from being untouched and unloved, although I don't profess to understand the mechanism. But I do think this element is one whose importance we should not underestimate."

An active lay leader in the Jewish Reconstructionist Movement, Jack also found warmth and support in his congregation. Knowing that the members of the synagogue were praying for his good health was deeply comforting to him. "There is something magical in the collective power of a group, some force larger than the sum of its components," he explains. "Knowing that a community of several hundred people is caring for you has a power, a force to lift you a little bit out of yourself.

"I believe prayers *do* change things, in that way, although as a Reconstructionist Jew I do not believe in the traditional idea of an Almighty with ears who can hear prayers and who intervenes in nature. Nor do I believe in a life after death in the ordinary sense that the soul passes through the pearly gates."

Jack has been chairman of his synagogue, and presently devotes a great deal of time to his duties as president of the National Federation of Reconstructionist Congregations. Since his graduation from law school, he has always worked for Jewish concerns. In 1973 he became administrator of the Board of Jewish Education of Greater New York. This dedication to Judaism, combined with his law degree, leads him to joke, "I'm on jury duty fifty-two weeks a year—that's jury spelled J-E-W-R-Y."

Since Jack's recovery from surgery, he has received no further treatment for cancer, although he has had periodic checkups with Dr. Cahan. While Jack has shown no further symptoms of cancer, four months after the operation he had a scare. Vacationing on Cape Cod with Faigal, he suddenly developed severe chest pains. The couple rushed back to New York, where Dr. Cahan examined Jack thoroughly. The tests showed no apparent cause for the sharp pains; the doctor concluded that internal adhesions, or even muscles, might have torn, and if that were the case, the stabbing pain should soon disappear. Within a week, it did.

Another incident, five years later, had Jack thinking, "Well, this is it. It's come back." After five years free of cancer, he suddenly began spitting up blood. He checked into the hospital in the middle of the night. The following day Dr. Cahan examined him and ordered a bronchoscopy; but this examination of Jack's lungs showed no tumorous cells. For ten days, Jack continued to cough up blood while every conceivable test was run, always with negative results. The tests included a sophisticated X ray called a bronchogram. For Jack, this was one of the worst ordeals he had ever gone through, since a chalky substance was inserted into his bronchia by means of a small slit in his throat—and the entire procedure had to be done while he was awake.

That test, too, showed that his lungs were clear of cancer. Gradually the volume of blood Jack coughed up decreased, until finally his sputum was clear. It was impossible to confirm the cause of this frightening symptom, but it may have been a sudden hemorrhage in lung tissue which finally healed itself.

Jack maintains a perspective on himself as a healthy man and has done so since the very beginning of his fight with cancer. In fact, as soon as he had thoroughly recovered from his surgery in 1965, he decided to exercise. When he went in for a routine physical a year after the operation, Dr. Cahan commented, "You're looking great. What are you doing to keep yourself in condition?"

"Well, I've been doing some pushups."

Cahan looked at him for a moment, and then said, "You're kidding."

"No," said Jack. "I wanted to get back in shape."

"Show me."

Jack got down on the floor of the office and began to do pushups. Cahan stopped him after half a dozen. "That's fantastic after such radical surgery!" he said. "Would you mind coming in sometime to demonstrate for some other physicians in a seminar?"

Jack, who had thought this was nothing special, agreed.

Two weeks later he stood in a conference room at Sloan-Kettering in front of some sixty physicians and medical students. "I'd like you to see what a cancer patient can do one year after thoracic surgery," Dr. Cahan told the group.

With that, Jack got down on the floor and did his pushups until he was stopped by Dr. Cahan.

He received a standing ovation.

Jack jogs two or three times a week at a nearby health club. This, too, he undertook on his own initiative, first asking Dr. Cahan whether it would be good for him. At first, toning the muscles was quite painful, and only rigorous self-discipline kept Jack going.

He admits that this self-discipline is the result of the simplest possible motivation—human vanity. "I'd like to think I take better care of myself because I had lung cancer," he says, "but perhaps that would be giving myself more credit than I deserve. I'm like many people; we get older, and we want to look younger. It's just plain vanity, and that's an honest answer."

Jack faithfully submits to an annual physical exam. In 1976 this routine exam saved his life. Jack had gone into Cahan's office feeling fine, with no symptoms of any kind to report. The doctor detected a pulse in a strange place, however; closer examination showed that it was an aneurysm pulsing in the aorta, which comes down from the heart into the body. A heart surgeon performed major surgery on Jack, installing a seven-inch piece of nylon tubing to replace the weakened section of aorta. "Now this," says Jack, "had nothing to do with cancer. And I had no symptoms. But if I hadn't gone in for that routine examination, that aorta could have burst and killed me." Again, Jack bounced back from major surgery. After a month he was back at work.

Jack views the life-threatening situations he has experienced as simply part of the whole process of living. "Life is life," he says with a shrug. "Cancer is always a threat, but so is the street. You never know when you might get mugged or run down by a car. And even if a person has cancer, he should be thinking about his future—and looking forward to it. Any of us can have an accident at any moment. Nobody has any guarantee of a secure existence in this world. In other words, there's always risk—but you have to go on living."

At age sixty-five, how has Jack been changed by his bout with cancer? "Naturally I have a different outlook on life today," he says. "I am sure trivialities bother me less. I don't let little irritants upset me, because I know they're simply not worth the emotional energy. It could be that my thinking has changed as a result of having cancer, and it could be the natural maturing process of the past seventeen years. I suspect that it's both."

Considering death, Jack says, "I never look upon my own impending death as a tragedy. I didn't fear death as a younger man, and I don't today.

"We all have to die. Death is an inevitable part of the whole life process. What really counts is how you make your departure from this world. If you can do it under happy auspices, friendly circumstances, if you go out in style, that's how to do it. In that way, dying should be like living: if you live in style, you ought to be ready to die in style.

"I hope to confront my death with courage. In facing cancer or any other such adversary, I believe we have an obligation to behave with dignity. I would hope to meet that situation like a man—like a righteous person who loves life."

5

OTTO GRAHAM

Otto Graham will long be remembered as one of America's greatest athletes. During his senior year, 1943–1944, at Northwestern, he was named All-American in both football and basketball—no other athlete has ever been named to both teams in a single season.

When Coach Paul Brown began putting together the Cleveland Browns, he signed Otto as his first player and quarterback. The Browns went on to play in title games for ten consecutive years, beginning in 1946—the ten-year period in which Otto played professional football—and to win the league championship seven out of those ten years. No other football team has ever approached the ten-year reign of the Cleveland Browns, and no one has ever doubted that Otto Graham was the team's superstar. The Professional Football Hall of Fame lists his quarterback statistics as football's all-time best.

Following his retirement from pro football, Otto served for several years as head coach and athletic director for the United States Coast Guard Academy. After three years as general manager and head coach of the Washington Redskins, he returned to the academy, where he is now athletic director.

Both as a quarterback and as a coach, Otto Graham has inspired thousands of young athletes and millions of fans. Today the legendary quarterback is in his sixties, but he continues to inspire large numbers of people, though his battle is no longer on the gridiron. It is a more important battle against a tougher opponent than he ever faced on the field—cancer.

To Otto Graham, cancer is just that—one more adversary, which must be faced like any other. A past Honorary Crusade Chairman of the American Cancer Society, he brings this message to large audiences all over the country, telling of his own bout with cancer and what he has learned from it. With the same direct style he brought to football, he talks frankly about cancer. At a recent Prudential Life Insurance convention, for instance, he addressed 1,700 sales agents and 800 managers in two separate talks. Near the end of each speech he asked for a show of hands: "Who has seen a doctor for a physical exam during the past year?"

The big ex-athlete looked out over the audience at the numerous people who had not raised their hands.

"To each of you who did not raise your hand," he said in his deep, vibrant voice, "I've got just one thing to say. You're a damn fool."

With the timing of a seasoned football player and a natural showman, Otto paused to let the message sink in. Then he added, "You people tell people like me to review our insurance program every year, study what's happened since last year and see what's changed. Well, practice what you preach! Review your health! The most important thing any of us has is our health. *You've got to get those annual physicals.* I have a tendency to procrastinate like the next guy. But I was lucky. I'm in the Coast Guard, and in the military you're required to get an annual physical. I had to get mine."

Even so, it was not through his physical in December 1977 that Otto's cancer was detected. He took the physical around Christmastime, when the cadets were home for the holidays

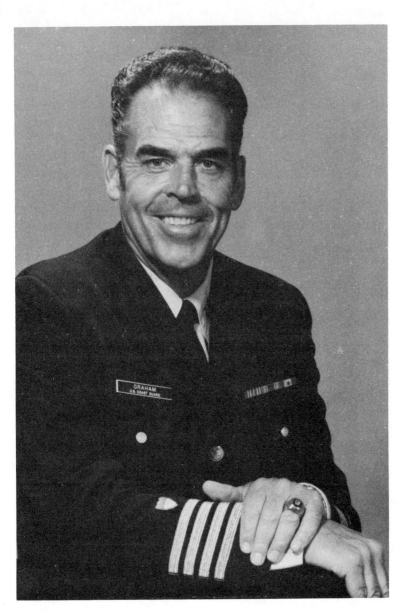

OTTO GRAHAM

and the hospital was less crowded. But, he admits, "Like so many guys, I skipped the proctoscopy . . . for the second year in a row."

Then, two months later, while doing some calisthenics, he felt twinges of pain in his tailbone. He ignored the pain for three days, thinking he had strained himself. Then he began to think about the fact that he had skipped the proctoscopy during his physical; and that his predecessor at the academy had died of cancer of the rectum. He made another appointment with the doctor.

The soreness Otto felt was a blessing in disguise. It was indeed muscle strain and nothing more—but the proctoscopy showed up something else. The doctor's face after the examination told Otto something was not right; so did the hushed conversation between the physician and an associate out in the hall.

When the doctor returned, Otto said, "Okay, I want you to give it to me straight. Is there anything wrong?"

The doctor hesitated and then replied, "There's an area that looks very suspicious. We're going to take a biopsy; we won't know anything until we get the biopsy report back."

Calmly Otto asked him, "What's your educated guess?"

"I would say there's a good chance you have cancer."

When the report came back, it confirmed the doctor's suspicion: Otto had cancer of the rectum. The doctor believed it had been detected early enough to save Otto's life but warned that until the operation it was impossible to tell how extensive the cancer might be. There was no way of knowing whether a colostomy would be necessary.

Surgery was scheduled at Bethesda Naval Hospital in Maryland. Otto was forced to cancel out of two golf tournaments that he was to play in Florida that March. He thought about delaying the operation until after the tournaments but decided against waiting.

Just before he went under the anesthetic he said, "Listen, Doc, if you have to do a colostomy, which side will it be on?"

"The left side," the doctor replied. "Colostomies are always on the left side."

"Good," said Otto. "I don't want it to interfere with my golf and tennis swing."

Still woozy from the effects of the anesthetic when the surgeon came into his room after the operation, Otto managed to say, "Well, Doc, tell me . . . can I still pass gas?"

"Yes, Otto," said the surgeon, "but not in the same way."

"So I've had a colostomy?" Otto asked. The doctor nodded.

If there was one thing ten seasons of pro football had taught the six-foot exquarterback, it was that when you're knocked down you get back up and keep going. The second day after his surgery he could be seen walking endlessly up and down the corridors of Bethesda Naval Hospital, pushing a little cart that held intravenous liquid, with the IV needle taped to his arm and the tube for the catheter concealed under his robe. A second tube was attached to his nose and led to his stomach.

But he wasn't on his feet very long. The next day Otto came down with a sudden fever. Since pneumonia was a real possibility, the temperature of 103 degrees alarmed the medical staff, who insisted that he cough and break up the phlegm in his lungs. Otto tried to do what they asked, but every attempt to cough brought on terrible pain. Holding a pillow tightly against his stomach did not help. Finally an orderly wheeled in a machine, and the doctor put a tube from the machine through Otto's other nostril and into his lungs, explaining, "This will make you cough."

The superathlete was so accustomed to pain that he never took novocain at the dentist's office. In his ten years as a quarterback, he had learned to ignore pain and keep going. In one game, for instance, his badly gashed jaw had been given twelve stitches during halftime. At the start of the third quarter, a bandaged Otto came running onto the field, to the surprise and delight of the fans. "You don't play football with your mouth," Otto explained at the time. "You play it with your arms and legs."

Now, for the first time in his life, he experienced a pain he could not handle. The machine did make him cough, some eight or ten times, and with a force and violence he had no control over. "It felt like my whole body exploded," he says somberly. "It was the worst pain I've ever experienced in my life, worse than any football injury. Believe me, I'll never forget it."

The coughing was effective, however. Within an hour, Otto's temperature dropped to 101 degrees, and then continued down. The same day a different machine was wheeled into his room. This one was something he could handle. He was told to suck in on a tube and fill his lungs with air, while watching the meter on the machine. The harder he inhaled, the higher the number he would see registered on the meter.

"They told me to do it hard enough to get up to number ten," he remembers, "and to do that ten times a day. That would keep my lungs clear. There was no way I wanted that coughing again. I got that meter up to twenty, and I did it twenty times a day. Believe me, I'd do anything to avoid *that* pain."

Instead Otto soon experienced a different kind of pain when he got a bad result on a CEA.*

"The normal range for this test is 0 to 5," he explains. "When my first blood count was 1, I thought, 'Hmm, that's good.' The next time I took the test, it was 2.5, and I thought, 'Oh my God, I'm going to die!' It was still in normal range—

---

* Carcinoembryonic antigen test is a blood test commonly given to cancer patients.

nevertheless, I was scared. I woke up in the middle of the night and couldn't stop worrying. I said to myself, 'Go to sleep, you fool,' but I lay awake the rest of the night.

"The third time I took the test, it went down to 1.7, and I slept well again. But then it jumped to 5.2! And I thought, 'Oh no, now I *know* I'm going to die!'"

Otto's fears were in fact unfounded—as he himself knew. Other tests were clear, and the CEA was not high enough to be alarming. Nevertheless, his fear was very real, and it resulted in a surprising appearance of pain. "I began to have all *kinds* of pains," he says, "and every little pain felt a hundred times worse than it really was. I was dying. And as soon as that count went back down, those pains went away. That's when I really learned how certain pains are mostly on the mind."

Before he left Bethesda, Otto talked to doctors there about follow-up treatment. Some advised chemotherapy and radiation. The chief medical officer thought it was not necessary, that the surgery had removed all the cancer. "If I were you, I'd have a wait-and-see attitude," he suggested. Otto decided to follow his advice.

With his wife, Beverly, Otto flew back to Connecticut, while their youngest son, David, drove the family car home. David had resigned his graduate assistantship at a Pennsylvania college, and his wife had resigned her job, so they could come to be with Otto and Beverly during his recovery. "The whole family was great," Otto says proudly. "We've got three children, two foster daughters, and twelve grandkids. They've all been wonderful."

Otto was home from the hospital and rested from the trip when David and his wife arrived with the car. David's greeting was, "Well, Dad, are you ready for some ping-pong?"

Otto beams. "Can you imagine? Here I am, I just had an operation two and a half weeks ago, and he challenges me to a game of ping-pong! See, we play some pretty good ping-pong, and he knows I like it. I said, 'Okay, you got yourself a game!'

"He said, 'Oh, hey Dad, I was just kidding.'

"And I said, 'They operated on my fanny and stomach, not my arms and eyes. Let's go.'"

During the game, Otto found he couldn't leap or lean for some shots. "But anything that came to me," he says, "I just put away. I won all three games. I couldn't do it again in a million years. But I have to say, it felt great. Fantastic."

Otto credits most of his rapid convalescence to the moral support he received from family and friends from all over the world. Over a hundred letters a day had been delivered to his hospital room. Several United States senators dropped by to visit, and Richard Nixon and Gerald Ford telephoned. Otto remembers the cards, calls, and visits with gratitude.

For the first few days that he was home, Otto made good progress and felt much better. Then, on the tenth day, he suffered an attack of stomach cramps, which became more intense every passing hour. He endured the pain until midnight, when he finally had to be taken to the academy's hospital.

Adhesions had strangled his bowels so that nothing could pass through. For two days the doctors tried unsuccessfully to get his system to function properly. Finally he was prepped for a second surgery.

Once again, Otto kissed Beverly goodbye and told her not to worry—the operation would be over in about two hours. It was just four weeks after the first operation, and the surgeon would cut through the fresh scar.

The operation was not as easy as Otto expected, however; it took five hours instead of two. Shaking his head a little, he explains, "They started sewing me up, did the inner layer, the muscles, and the skin, and then realized they couldn't find a sponge! So they opened me up again. And *then* it wasn't inside me. They found it eventually. In the meantime, my wife was worried to death. So even doctors can make a mistake," he concludes with a shrug.

Two weeks later, Otto was transferred to the local hospital, Lawrence Memorial, where he remained for the next four weeks. His second surgery was more devastating than the first. During this hospital confinement, he lost forty-five pounds and was down to 172, which he had not weighed since his freshman year in high school. "I was feeling just awful," he admits. "In fact, I had doubts about whether I was going to make it. During this time, they must have X-rayed me three hundred times. I figure those X rays had to make me sterile. But at my age, who cares?"

Unlike during his first hospitalization, Otto now found that visits from friends and relatives were a burden. "I was really sick, and wanted to be left alone," he says. "I just didn't have the strength—physical or mental—to see people. Even with my family, I would sometimes find myself thinking, 'I wish to hell they'd go home and leave me alone.' I was emotionally exhausted, and I wasn't up to making conversation. If people do visit, even relatives, they should stay just a short time; to a sick person, ten or fifteen minutes can seem like an eternity— especially when the next guy stays that long, and the next, and the one after him. God! I had times when I'd had it up to here with visitors, and just wanted to be left alone. Just wanted to lie there by myself."

The adhesions that brought Otto into the hospital a second time had caused a blockage so that his colostomy didn't work at all—his body was not eliminating. Even after the second operation, this continued to be a problem, and he was given a medication to soften his bowels and advised to drink plenty of water. "With the catheter in me, I felt like I had to urinate every ten seconds," he says, "and I was drinking less water to avoid that. I know now that that was a mistake. But finally, after six weeks, something came loose and I was in business. The colostomy began to operate."

During the difficult six weeks of hospital confinement Otto's thoughts wavered between a fear of dying and a desire to get well enough to play in the Bogey Busters. This celebrity golf tournament in Dayton, Ohio, was something he had looked forward to immensely. Happily, he got out of the hospital in time to make it. "When I first got out on the course, it was rough," he says. "During the three weeks before the tournament, I practiced four times. I was so weak, I was shanking putts, and I couldn't hit the ball very far. By the day of the tournament I learned to compensate for my weakness by using a five iron to reach the green from 150 yards out, instead of an eight iron. Actually, I played better golf. I was more accurate that day in Dayton than I'd been in the past. I was teamed up with Gerry Ford, Don Shula, Boots Randolph, the saxophone player, and Jim MacDonald, current president of General Motors—and we won. It was a great time. I didn't want to miss it, and I didn't miss it."

Otto's five handicap in golf proves that he is still a good golfer. His tennis game is also back in top form. He feels he is not physically debilitated in any way from his bout with cancer. "The doctors told me I would be able to do everything I ever did before," he says. "I believed them, and they were right." In addition to golf and tennis, Otto does calisthenics for ten minutes every morning, and carefully watches his diet—although he admits to a weakness for desserts. However, he is only two pounds over his playing weight as a pro quarterback. This has been achieved, he does not hesitate to say, through sheer self-discipline. "Most athletes gain weight when they stop playing because they're used to burning up so many calories as pros. They've got to realize that they don't need the same intake once they quit playing," he says.

Otto believes that pro sports gave him more than just self-discipline. "An athlete has to deal with adversity all the time. For one thing, there's injury. You get a broken ankle and end up with a cast on your leg and a crutch. Or you get a shoulder separation. That's all part of the sport. You've got to accept it. Adversity helps build people, and when it's a fact of life that occurs constantly, you learn to deal with it. I feel sorry for the person who lives, so to speak, with a silver spoon in his mouth, and never faces adversity. When it finally does hit him—and it will, sooner or later—he doesn't know how to cope."

Otto claims that as a fiercely competitive pro football player he experienced blows more devastating than the discovery that he had cancer. "Sure, it was traumatic to find out I had cancer. But compared to losing the championship . . . You see, I played in ten championships in a row, and got so psyched up for those games! We lost three of those ten, and each time we lost I sunk to an all-time low. There's nothing like it. People may not understand the feeling, but to a pro athlete, it's his life not just a game. I have to say in all honesty, when I found out about my cancer I was nowhere near the low that I experienced when we lost those championships. When you lose you're at rock bottom. But in either case—a lost championship or a bout with cancer—you've got to pick up the pieces and figure out how to go on from there."

This message is something Otto brings to every speech he makes. "I've had a colostomy," he says. "I know some people think, 'Oh my God, it's going to ruin my life!' But that's not true nowadays. It's not like the old days when you had to stay at home, lie in bed all day. There's no lack of mobility anymore. Believe me, this is something you can learn to live with. Sure, you have to go through cleaning it every so often and all that. So what? That's nothing. As long as the cancer's gone, you're doing fine."

Otto stresses the importance of humor. "Often I make a

joke of my cancer. It's my nature, my way. I can't do a damn thing about my colostomy. I've got it, and I can't change that fact, so I make the best of it. Joke about it. Why not?"

He is likely to tell an audience, "If I could change and go back to the old way of elimination—you know, I wouldn't do it.

"Stop and think. Now that I've had a colostomy, I will never have to worry about hemorrhoids. I don't have to worry about finding a bathroom. You know, go down the hall, turn left, then right . . . Or suppose you stop at a restaurant or a filling station to use the toilet. *I* don't have to do that—no more worry about dirty toilet seats. No more bedpans in the hospital, and you know how uncomfortable bedpans are. No more proctoscopes or rectal thermometers. Suppose I have to pass gas. Well, I do have to worry about that. I don't have a sphincter muscle around my colostomy, so I can't control it. All I do when I pass gas, then, is turn to my wife and say, 'What did you say, dear?'"

Many people have stopped Otto after meetings to thank him for making a colostomy something they can joke about instead of something they feel compelled to hide. Women have said that seeing him make light of a colostomy—an operation which means a serious change in the functioning of one's body—has made it easier for them to accept the loss of a breast to cancer.

With a boyish grin, he says, "There's a time to be serious and a time to have fun. You've got to fight cancer damn seriously, but you've got to keep your sense of humor, too."

Fellow volunteers of the local American Cancer Society chapter in Wallingford got a taste of Otto's sense of humor on one occasion. Before this meeting, a friend of his was joking with him about her double mastectomy, the cost of the operation and of the prosthetic bra, and so forth. When she got up to speak, she felt encouraged to talk as Otto does, of the "advantages" of having a double mastectomy. "I can be anybody I want to with my falsies. I can even be Jayne Mansfield if I want to."

Otto couldn't resist heckling. "Hey, Falsie LaRue," he yelled, "the *least* you can do is get 'em on straight. You got one dangling!" Then he bounded up on the stage and, to the delight of the group and the speaker, proceeded to straighten them out.

"It broke the place up. She laughed harder than anyone," Otto reports.

"I know one thing, when you're laughing and having a good time, you're not going to be so conscious of hurting. And another thing: Stress and negative thinking can harm your health. So you've got to enjoy life. Look for the best. Have a good time."

Despite his usually positive attitude, even Otto Graham has his occasional bad times. It is difficult to get him to talk about them, but he will admit, "I'm afraid of cancer. Cancer is an adversary I take very seriously. I make light of it, but don't let that fool you. If my blood tests aren't good, like I said, that scares me. In fact, every time I go in for those tests, I worry until I get the results. I think about those good times out on the golf course and visits to Florida, I think about my wife, my kids, those beautiful grandkids. . . . I'm not afraid of dying; we all have to die . . . but . . . "

His eyes glisten for a moment, and then with a little shake of his head he moves into a different mood. "See," he says earnestly, "pretty soon I'll be able to retire. And that's *another* good thing about this colostomy—it makes me eligible for 100 percent disability. That's tax-free income! If I die," and now his eyes are again bright with a joke, "if I die before I get to take advantage of this tax-free retirement income, I am going to be mad for all eternity!

"I'm enjoying life so much, just the way it is for me right now," he says. "I just want to keep on living." The sun-tanned man dressed in a short-sleeved Coast Guard officer's uniform pauses to reflect, looking out the window of his office in the academy's athletic department. The view is of the bay of the picturesque Thames River, where several Coast Guard vessels sway back and forth with the tide. It's springtime, and the New England hillside across the bay is very green and peaceful. Finally Otto says, "You know, when you have cancer, you learn something very valuable. You learn to live each and every day. You learn to enjoy it while you've got it.

"When my wife picked me up to take me home that second time I was in the hospital, it was early spring. The leaves were coming out, the grass was getting green, there were flowers everywhere.

"It's eight miles from the hospital to our house, and I've driven that road hundreds of times, but I never saw anything so beautiful in my life. I just soaked in the sight of those flowers, the grass, the leaves. I suppose I'd always been too doggone busy to really see. I was so wound up in my everyday life that I didn't appreciate the real beauty around me. I do now."

Leaning back in his chair, he says in a soft voice, "My wife and I have been blessed all our lives. We've really only experienced one misfortune. That was when Stevie died."

Years ago, Otto and Beverly went to the West Coast for a Rose Bowl game. While they were there, they received a telephone call; their six-week-old son, Stevie, had died—an inexplicable crib death. Many years later, Otto's voice is heavy and slow when he talks of this. "It was the saddest thing in our lives," he says simply. "When we buried him, for some reason I put a couple of pennies on the grave. I don't know why. I'm not superstitious, but I just did it. Ever since that time it seems that I'm always finding pennies. It's incredible how many I find, and in the oddest places. It's happened too often for me to think it's a coincidence. And every time, I feel like I hear Stevie saying, 'It's okay, I'm with you, Dad.'"

Otto attended church every Sunday as a youngster; his mother was a church organist. He is not a regular churchgoer today, but is a firm believer. "I don't think you have to go to church every Sunday to be a good Christian," he says. "I live a good Christian life, and I believe in the Christian philosophy. Now, when I was in bad shape with cancer, I didn't ask God to save me. In my prayers I said, 'If I make it, I'm going to be a better person and be more helpful to society.' And I have tried to do that."

As the 1980 Honorary Crusade Chairman of the American Cancer Society, Otto helped others survive what he himself survived. "I know that I have motivated some people to get a physical. If only one has been saved from cancer, then it's all been worthwhile.

"I've been lucky all my life. I was lucky, in the first place, to be born to a good Christian family. I've been lucky to be married nearly forty years to a woman who's been a wonderful wife and a fine mother. I was blessed with the God-given coordination to be an athlete. I was lucky to play football under Paul Brown, who was as good a coach as ever coached the game. And I've been very lucky to be in a position to speak out and reach a lot of people. I'm lucky to be alive and able to share my joy with others."

6

PHYLLIS LOEFF

In July 1978 Phyllis Loeff was just getting her life back in order after a traumatic and bizarre accident. The previous fall, as she was walking along a pedestrian passageway toward her car, a truck behind her suddenly backed up, rapidly picked up speed, struck her, knocked her down, and ran her over.

With her pelvis and legs crushed, Phyllis spent months in the hospital, not sure she would ever walk again. She was released to convalesce at home. With physical therapy and the use of a cane, she was walking again by the following April and able to resume seeing patients in her private psychiatric practice.

Phyllis had started her practice in 1969, twenty years after her graduation from medical school. When she had married Harold Loeff, a gynecologist, she had opted for a large family and devoted herself to raising their four children. During those years she used her medical background in community work with the American Red Cross, the local public schools, and charitable organizations. In 1966 Phyllis resumed her studies, and in 1969 she finished her residency in psychiatry.

Soon she had built a solid practice, working out of her home in Highland Park, an affluent suburb of Chicago.

The freakish truck accident had put the robust woman out of commission for nearly six months. By midsummer 1978 she had regained her former energy, although she was still dependent on a cane and involved in physical therapy. She was thankful that she had survived the devastating trauma to her body as well as she had. But one evening, rubbing her neck to ease tension, Phyllis felt a lump. "I wasn't looking for anything," she says, "but I felt something the size of an almond. As a physician, I immediately knew it wasn't supposed to be there."

For Phyllis, getting a second opinion was exceptionally easy: she asked her husband to feel the lump. His reaction, calm and noncommittal, was a dead giveaway. "I can always tell what he's thinking," Phyllis says. "If he says nothing, except that I should see another doctor, that tells me there's something remarkable about it. If there weren't, he would tell me not to worry and discuss it with me as one physician to another." Harold suggested another opinion. The next evening a good friend, Dr. Sidney Black, turned up at the house and said to Phyllis, "I want to see what this is all about."

When he had palpated the lump thoughtfully, he said, "Well, my dear, we'll have to do a biopsy."

Phyllis's reaction was calm. She knew the almond-sized lump could have been the result of any number of things. She was not very concerned, because she felt no pain, no symptoms of any kind. She comments, "That lack of symptoms points up the importance of self-examination—as the American Cancer Society is always telling people."

The following day, July 6, Phyllis went to Highland Park Hospital, where Sidney Black, chairman of surgery, did a biopsy. The outpatient operation was performed under local anesthetic. As a result, Phyllis had the unusual experience of suspecting the results of the biopsy even as it was being performed. Watching Dr. Black's eyes, and the quiet, sober faces around her, she knew there was a serious problem. Without comment, they took a frozen biopsy, and Phyllis was wheeled back to her room.

Before the morning was over, her husband came to her room. The results of the biopsy were in. He said quietly, "Well, it's thyroid." Phyllis knew beyond a doubt that he meant cancer of the thyroid.

Again, the physician-patient took the news calmly. She knew that thyroid carcinoma is not as life threatening and fast moving as many forms of cancer. Moreover, "It's not my style to get hysterical," she comments. "I think part of that is my medical background. A physician has to be courageous and maintain equanimity and poise about this sort of thing. I wouldn't say I was stoic; but I was quiet."

The truck accident now seemed like only a dress rehearsal for this new threat to her life. While double blows of this kind often lead people to ask, "Why me?" Phyllis says, "Why not me?" In her soft, level voice she explains, "I work with innocent people who, for one reason or another, have had bad luck of all sorts. In this world we continually see innocent people encounter very unfortunate circumstances, and there is no real reason for this. So it didn't occur to me to ask, 'Why me?' 'Why not me?' is as plausible a response."

Even so, Phyllis faced the difficult fact that, although she was a physician, she could not predict the extent to which this thyroid carcinoma would interrupt her life. She could accept the idea that she would undergo procedures she dreaded and that her body would be irrevocably changed by this. It was more difficult to keep from wondering just how much her life would be changed.

Because cancer of the thyroid is slow moving, Phyllis was able to schedule surgery almost three weeks away, giving her time to put her affairs in order. This was perhaps more im-

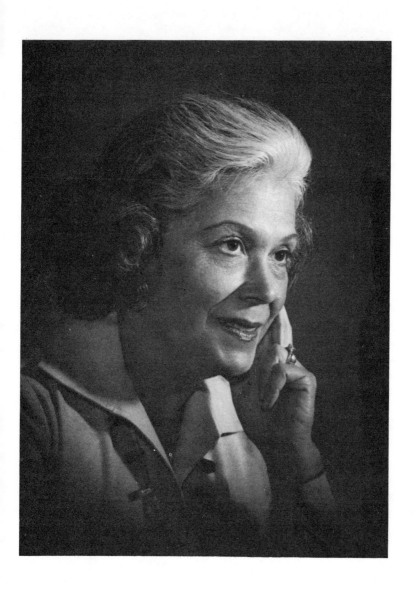

PHYLLIS LOEFF

portant in her profession than in some, since it meant telling all her patients that she would not see them again until after Labor Day. The analytically oriented psychotherapy she practices does not suffer as much from such an interruption as some forms of therapy, and she was able to reschedule patients without giving a detailed explanation of her reason. Since many psychiatrists take their vacations during August, there were few questions asked.

During this time Phyllis learned a sad truth: her thyroid carcinoma was the result of well-intentioned medical treatment many years ago. She explains that during the early forties, a distinguished dermatologist used X rays for treating acne. This was also a popular method for shrinking enlarged tonsils in children. The X-ray treatments were phenomenally successful. After the treatment, the patient developed a skin flush for a day or two and then, almost miraculously, the acne disappeared. "It was painless," Phyllis remembers, "and the doctor was a lovely man who believed he was using the most advanced kind of treatment. My family took me to him with equal trust that they were getting the best possible medical care for me."

In recent years, however, Michael Reese Hospital has attempted to locate every person who received the innovative treatments, for a high number of them have developed cancer of the thyroid. Fortunately, this treatment was not widely used. In Chicago, however, there are a number of people with thyroid carcinoma who were given what seemed at the time like the best possible medical treatment for their teenage acne or enlarged tonsils.

As she confronted her operation, Phyllis was aware of the delicacy of this particular surgery. While her thyroid and lymph glands would have to be removed, the parathyroid glands would be carefully isolated, since they are essential for the metabolism of calcium. Furthermore, there was a risk that the innervation to the larynx, which winds around the thyroid gland, might be disturbed. If it were, the result could be a permanent loss of voice.

For her surgeon, Phyllis chose a man of great reputation, Dr. Tapas Dasgupta, born in India, trained at Sloan-Kettering, and now head of the oncology department at the University of Illinois. "He is one of the finest surgeons in the world for this kind of operation," she says. "He can literally take a person apart and put them back together again—after removing all the tumerous tissue he can find. So it gave me great comfort to know I was in his hands." It was also comforting to know that Sidney Black would attend the surgery and that her husband, Harold, was waiting nearby, able to respond as a physician if any decisions were necessary during the surgery. "I have enormous respect for both Dr. Dasgupta and Dr. Black," she says. "But as a physician I was also aware of the fact that anything can happen during a cancer operation. You never know what you will find."

What the surgeon did find was a chain of cancerous lymphatic glands in Phyllis's neck, which he removed; he did not remove any muscle tissue at all. When she opened her eyes after the surgery, the first thing Phyllis did was say, "Hi."

"I was glad to hear my own voice!" she says. "I did lose my ability to sing because of the surgery, and I loved to sing. But I have good memories of singing, and I am very grateful for the success of the operation."

Despite her medical background, Phyllis was not prepared for the size of the incision on her neck. "I felt like the Scarecrow in *The Wizard of Oz*," she says. Because the drainage is changed, the left side of her face is slightly puffy, too. These things, however, "blur into unimportance in comparison to what could have happened."

Even so, the cancer and the operation had a dramatic effect on Phyllis emotionally. While she had anticipated a difference in the way she looked, she was not entirely prepared for the change in "the wholeness, or integrity, of my body. I had a scar to remind me of my vulnerability. And that disruption in the smoothness of my skin kept telling me there was something very serious underneath that had been removed."

She is now required to take synthetic thyroid every day, since her body no longer produces this key endocrine. Thyroid is essential to metabolism and, therefore, to life itself. "If I were shipwrecked and had no thyroid medication," Phyllis explains, "I would eventually become more and more cretinous, and finally die."

Thyroid medication, commonly prescribed for people with sluggish thyroid glands, has no side effects. Phyllis needs to be concerned with it only twice a year, when she has blood samples taken for analysis to make sure her metabolic levels are adequate. Her operation changed her physical therapy regime, and neck exercises were added, since elasticity and mobility can be reduced after neck surgery. Before Labor Day she was seeing some of her patients, and by mid-September she had gone back to her regular routine.

No chemotherapy was prescribed for Phyllis's malignancy, with the exception of a single high dose of radioactive iodine. This medication, a small, potent drink of what looks like clear water, is thought to move through the circulatory system to seek out remaining cancerous thyroid cells in the body and destroy them.

Once every year Phyllis takes a far smaller dose of this radioactive iodine for several days in preparation for her annual CAT scan. This dose is not intended to kill tumerous tissue but to mark thyroid cells so they are visible to the scan, which would otherwise show them as hot spots. To prepare for the scan, Phyllis must endure the unpleasant consequences of discontinuing her thyroid medication for several weeks. The result of this is that she begins to feel sluggish and fatigued, and gains weight through fluid retention. "It's a tough time for me," she admits. "The chemical reaction makes me somewhat spacy—and depressed. It's more than just a case of the blahs; it's a sad feeling. It's . . . not pleasant. But I'm willing to live through it because I feel it's necessary."

Once the scan is completed, Phyllis begins her thyroid medication again, and in a week or two her metabolism is back to normal. "All in all, I have to consent to be sick for about five weeks every year—just to make sure I'm not ill." But, she adds, "this is one of the sequels of this disease, and it's something I accept without much complaint."

While her endocrinologist strongly believed the regular CAT scans were essential, Phyllis's surgeon just as strongly disagreed. He insisted that he had removed every bit of cancer and that the radioactive iodine might damage Phyllis's lung tissue in the future. He also noted that thyroid cancer is very slow growing, so that he believed such frequent monitoring through this test was not necessary.

Phyllis found this put her in a difficult position, with two competent doctors in total disagreement and each assuring her that his advice was correct. "I felt caught in the middle," she explains, "because I respected both doctors equally. My husband and I discussed this matter with several of our colleagues, and they, too, disagreed. Finally I decided that since my endocrinologist was the specialist who had worked with the radioactive iodine, I would follow his recommendation. It's tough to be a patient who has to make a decision of this magnitude, and only time will tell whether I made the right decision.

"Here I am—a physician myself, married to a physician. What's a layman supposed to do in this kind of situation? Carcinoma is one of those disorders where the treatment may be different according to whom you ask. And the patient can frequently be caught in the middle. With all that I knew, I still felt the difficulty of being a patient."

Although deciding on treatment when doctors disagree can

be very difficult, Phyllis believes that every patient should seek a second opinion and that doctors should encourage this. "I know I would never want the responsibility of being the only one to work with a serious disorder," she says. "I think it's just good medicine to have it confirmed, not by an associate or friend but by someone else, perhaps from a teaching center."

Phyllis has an unusual perspective on this issue, since she is a patient, an M.D., and a psychiatrist. Patients who seek confirming opinions, she believes, have more confidence, and this can make treatment more effective. She also believes in the importance of sensitive communication between patient and physician. "Part of the skill and art of medicine is for a physician to know how much information to offer, and when. Certainly a patient should be informed about what to expect so he isn't completely overwhelmed by what happens. At the same time, the doctor should avoid making it gruesome. With medications, for instance, the patient should have some understanding of possible side effects, but this should be presented in such a way, and at such a time, that it isn't frightening."

The consequences for a patient of being uninformed, Phyllis feels, can be grave. "He may later have a bitterness, a feeling that he didn't know all the alternatives. He may feel he has not been respected. It's not a matter of how a patient feels before surgery or chemotherapy but of how he feels afterward which is most important. Usually there is not much time to debate surgery for cancer. But when the surgery is over and done with, the issue must be dealt with. The patient has time to think, and often he thinks, 'Why didn't I know? I would have felt better.' Because he was not informed, he feels depersonalized, dehumanized."

In the long run, Phyllis believes, cancer patients are stronger and better able to deal with their illness when they have been given the power to make choices and been kept fully informed. "I recommend that a physician put the cards on the table beforehand; this helps to prevent negative feelings after surgery, when the patient is even more vulnerable, and needs to recuperate and get back on his feet. It's a very poor situation when a patient is asking, 'Why wasn't this done instead of that? Why wasn't I told about this?' That doubt is negative, and impedes recovery."

The gray-haired psychiatrist adds that honesty does not mean tactlessness. Even when there is little or no hope of survival, a physician should not announce to a patient, "I'm sorry, but there is no hope." Since it takes time for an individual to adjust to a fatal illness, she suggests that it is more comforting if a physician initially says something like, "We'll do everything we can, but it's serious."

When the symptoms of cancer become so serious as to be undeniable, Phyllis believes it is important to help patients prepare for death. Because of this belief, she is a member of the Medical Advisory Committee of the Hospice at Highland Park Hospital. This is one of many such special units that have sprung up around the country in the past two decades or so, devoted to the care and treatment of those who have life-threatening illnesses (a term which is often a euphemism for terminal illness). Highland Park's hospice shelters many cancer patients, as well as others who may have kidney failure, neurological wasting diseases, etc. A model facility, it is one of a handful licensed by the state of Illinois and therefore eligible for federal funding. "It is a remarkable unit," Phyllis says proudly. "The nurses are specially trained, and every effort is made to maintain the patient's dignity at all times. Family members are permitted to visit any time of the day or night. And, above all, the emphasis is always placed on the patient's comfort."

In her practice, as well as at hospice, Phyllis has often dealt with the issue of how people can prepare for death. She has observed that when a life-threatening illness strikes, people usually want to discuss unfinished business with those who are close to them—and this is an important aspect of "getting one's affairs in order."

"Anger may exist," she says softly, "or there may be certain disappointments—for instance, between a parent and a grown child. People often need to say to a family member, 'I knew this happened, and I want you to know I knew it. It's all right.' They may need to say, 'I'm facing a serious operation, and afterwards, who knows what might happen? I want you to know I love you. . . . I want to settle this old problem with you. . . . I want to talk about who I want to have what.' This kind of discussion with loved ones is good for anyone who contemplates death. It may be an emotional workout, and it should be the patient's choice whether to do this, since not everybody prefers to clear the decks in this fashion. But it's better than keeping guilt and frustrations pent up, and in the long run the patient benefits."

As a cancer patient and psychiatrist, Phyllis has a rare insight into dealing with life-threatening illnesses. Consequently, other physicians on occasion refer patients to her. She does not always talk about her own health history with clients, especially if it does not seem relevant, but she has developed a special empathy for clients who have suffered serious injury or illness.

"I think they know how I feel," she says, her hazel eyes soft and thoughtful. "They know I'm not condescending. Often there are things they don't need to explain· in great detail, because I understand. There's no question that these things are different when you experience them firsthand, although a competent psychiatrist who has never experienced such a problem can certainly transcend that limitation." With a slight gesture toward the cane that leans against the wall of her office, she adds, "They know I've experienced the pain, the trauma, the debilitating effects of surgery, and the concern over health. I've had the wear and tear they've had. In the field of psychiatry, we refer to the narcissistic injury or illness; that is when one's body has been deformed or scarred or something else beyond normal aging, when an insult to the integrity of your own self has occurred. Such a thing does alter your self-image and other people's response to you, and necessitates a major adjustment. This is true for people who suffer from cancer, as well as those who have faced any kind of major illness or physical injury."

Her own illness, Phyllis found, has changed her relationships and sharpened her perspective. She is now more likely to react openly and directly to problems. "It's not that I've become dominating or interfering," she says. "I wasn't that sort of individual before, and I'm still not. But when I speak about something I care about, I'm more adventurous and more explicit in what I say. I have more courage to come out and speak my piece. That may mean saying, 'I'm afraid what you're doing might mean trouble for you,' or it may mean saying, 'I'm so glad for this.' It's not just negative, but also very positive; it works both ways. When I am happy, I am deeply happy. When I am pleased, I am very pleased. I am *so* encouraging to the people I care about, and I think in this regard the kind of support I am capable of giving them today is far greater than it was before."

Her accident and illness left Phyllis far less able to be physically active, and therefore they created more time for deep thought. The thyroid carcinoma has also given her a sense of the preciousness of life, since she believes that, realistically, some years will be subtracted from the end of her life. She credits this awareness for her greater assertiveness in reaching out to others. "It's not that I'm dogmatic," she says, "because I know my opinion may be wrong. It's rather a matter of wanting to share my thoughts with others so they may benefit in some way.

"I've become a very forthright person, and I'm not embarrassed to say to someone, 'I love you.' I get great pleasure from encouraging my family, friends, and patients to be aggressive, to be courageous, to take chances, to risk trying new things. I believe it's far better to fail than not to have the courage to at least try. And I try to share this philosophy with others."

This need to be useful and helpful is something Phyllis obviously felt long before her illness. But she is definite in her conviction that it is an attitude which has heightened since she faced cancer. "I wouldn't recommend what I've gone through as a way of improving everyday life," she says, smiling. "But you do have a certain zest for life when you know how precious it is, and how fragile it can be."

7

BEVERLY HALL

On December 5, 1979, Beverly Hall started her new job, as office manager and accounting supervisor for the Spring Manufacturing Company. "I can't tell you how thrilled I'd been to land this job," she says. "It was perfect—it was everything I wanted."

With the new job, the thirty-five-year-old wife and mother felt good about her life. After fifteen years of marriage, Beverly was comfortably adjusted to her role as wife of a Baptist minister and mother of two sons and a daughter. Now that their youngest son was in school, she felt free to find work she enjoyed, and hoped to save for the children's college education.

Beverly was excited about her new job, but surprised that she found the work so tiring. When she thought it over, however, it seemed only logical. The Halls had moved the previous year from Flint, Michigan, to Farmington, a suburb of Detroit. Now that Joe's church was in the process of relocating, they were moving again to a new home. With all that and the Christmas holidays coming, it was only natural to be tired.

Another thing that surprised her was her sudden, peculiar

tendency to bruise. For no apparent reason she developed large bruises on her legs, some of them the size of pancakes. Beverly could not remember bumping into things. At first Joe joked with her about them. "Be more careful. People are going to think I'm beating my wife, and that doesn't look good—especially for a minister."

After a few days, however, his concern grew over both the bruises and Beverly's extreme fatigue. When she told him she could hardly find the energy to drive home from work, he urged her to see John Cox, the family doctor. On a Wednesday after work she did so.

Dr. Cox examined Beverly and took a blood sample. Although this was an ordeal for her, since she had a long-entrenched fear of needles, she was almost too tired to complain. The next morning Dr. Cox called to tell Beverly that the blood report was "not good," and that he had sent the results to Providence Hospital in nearby Southfield for Dr. David Leichtman to look at. He asked Beverly to come in that afternoon with Joe, so that he could talk to both of them.

The family doctor was almost in tears as he faced Beverly and Joe in his office later that day. Gently he told them that Dr. Leichtman, who was both an oncologist and a hematologist, had confirmed his own suspicion—Beverly had leukemia. He explained that leukemia could be either acute or chronic, and that the latter type was far less critical. Beverly listened, not entirely shocked, remembering that her family had a history of cancer.

Dr. Cox told the young parents that Dr. Leichtman wanted Beverly admitted to the hospital immediately. For over an hour, the Halls waited in his office for a call confirming that a hospital bed was available. Finally word came that no bed would be available until morning. Dr. Cox told Joe, "Take her straight home, no stop, and promise me you'll put her right to bed." Bev's bruises were caused by low platelet counts, he explained, and those low counts meant that any cut

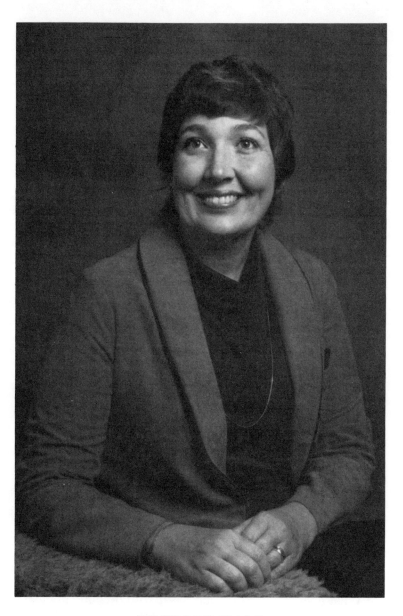

BEVERLY HALL

or bump could result in dangerous excessive bleeding, either internal or external. Carefully, Joe drove home, took Beverly into the house, and made sure she was safely tucked in bed. It was to be her last night in her own bed for many months.

The next morning Dr. Leichtman met the Halls in the emergency room of Providence Hospital. Beverly's impression of the specialist was favorable; he seemed "concerned, but also direct and professional." He explained that he had to take a sample of bone marrow to complete his diagnosis of Beverly's condition. The test was the first painful shock of the day. It entailed drilling a tiny hole in her backbone and using a special needle to extract a small chip of bone. After the test Beverly joined Joe in Dr. Leichtman's office.

"We need to establish right now what kind of relationship you'd like to have with me," he said to them. "Do you want to know everything, all the details? Or do you want to know the minimum?"

"Absolutely everything," they agreed.

Dr. Leichtman nodded, and then explained that Beverly had acute myelocytic leukemia, originating in the bone marrow rather than the lymph glands. "Most patients with acute leukemia," he said, "die before they ever get into remission."

Beverly took in the words but somehow could not connect them to herself. She had understood his diagnosis intellectually; at this point, the meaning of it for her life had not sunk in.

The doctor went on to describe the necessary treatment. Beverly must be put into isolation immediately, since she had virtually no immune defenses, and she must begin a program of chemotherapy.

"You're not going to like it," the physician said straightforwardly. "And you're likely to be confined to this hospital for a very long time. Furthermore, despite everything we can do, it's possible the disease will never reach remission."

"What does that mean?" Joe asked with hesitation.

"We need four or five months of treatment to get her into

remission. We may not get the time we need. If we're successful and we can achieve remission, then Beverly will have some time."

"How much time?" Joe asked.

"There's no way of predicting that."

The shocked couple tried to absorb this as Dr. Leichtman turned to the question of chemotherapy. The Halls had said they wanted to know everything; he described the probable side effects of the treatment he was recommending: extensive nausea; ulcerated sores on the mouth, esophagus, bowels, and rectum; loss of hair. For the first several weeks she would receive intravenous medication constantly through a machine by her bed. Because Beverly was immune-depressant, she would have to be in isolation in the hospital. She was extremely open to infection of any kind, and she was allergic to certain antibiotics and drugs, so she must be carefully protected from germs. Nobody would enter her room without donning a sterile gown, rubber gloves, and a mask. The children would not be able to visit.

Beverly sat silent, thinking of the life she had built. The new job, the new house, the children, the upcoming Christmas holidays—everything now seemed distant and irrelevant. All her dreams were shattered.

"I don't want any medication," she said. "I'm not hurting, and I'm not afraid of dying. All that sounds . . . like something I don't want to go through. Why should I suffer like that if this leukemia is going to kill me anyway?"

Dr. Leichtman stood up and walked to the door. "I'm going to leave for a while and give you a chance to talk this over with your husband."

After he left, Beverly and Joe sat silent for a few minutes, holding hands. Tears began to well up in Beverly as she thought about what she was facing.

And she thought about her children. She remembered her own childhood with a chronically ill parent. Her mother had suffered an almost constant string of health problems, complicated by a weak heart. She had had a tumor removed from a breast, had gone through major gynecological problems, and had had her gall bladder, one kidney, and part of the other kidney removed. Through all this, the young girl had hurt unbearably with fear of losing her mother. "I could remember that so vividly," Beverly says, "and I didn't want my children to go through it. It had been so bad for me as a child that at times I felt forsaken by God.

"As I thought about all of this, I believed that if I died, I would have peace. I would live with the Lord, and everything would be okay. I could handle the thought of dying a lot better than the thought of being really sick. When it comes to pain, I've always been a big baby, and I was scared silly of hypodermic needles. I was what you'd call a fraidy cat. But my feelings were very real. And after he told me what I'd have to go through, and still not live very long, I was terrified."

Beverly saw through her tears that Joe was crying, too. As the two clasped hands, she looked at him, trusting and waiting for his guidance. Finally, Joe said, "Honey, I will never lose you, no matter what happens. Whether you're here or in heaven, I'll always love you dearly and know that you're with me. But I need you here. I need you to fight. You have to fight, if not for yourself, then for me and the children. Please." Beverly knew she would make every effort to survive, not for herself, but for those who loved her.

When Dr. Leichtman returned, Beverly told him she had decided to have the chemotherapy. Joe kissed her and reluctantly left, to take the children to their school Christmas programs that night. Beverly went to the radiology department for a chest X ray, and then to the private room reserved for her.

That night she lay alone, listening to the quiet sounds of the hospital. She slept far less than she had the night before.

At 7:00 the next morning a doctor came to her room to administer her first medication. Beverly had never had an IV before, and the size of the needle alarmed her. As the doctor prepared the medication, she remembered a shot she had received many years before, when she and Joe were traveling across the country and she became ill. They stopped in a small town in the Arizona desert and went to a tiny hospital, where an injection was prescribed. Beverly's fear was so great that it was a struggle for Joe and a strong nurse to hold her still enough to receive the injection. "I nearly panicked again, but then I thought of the children. There would be a lot of unpleasant things in this whole experience, and the children were going to be watching me, like I watched my mom when I was little. I didn't want them to live with the same images and feelings I'd had as a child; I had felt so guilty when my mom suffered. I made up my mind that my children wouldn't go through that. So I would just have to adjust to these needles." This brand of courage had never been Beverly's strong suit. Nevertheless, frightened and in pain, she cooperated with the doctor, and the IV was installed.

The worst of Beverly's fears came true. She had nearly every possible side effect from the massive doses of chemotherapy. She vomited for hours. Her allergic reactions to the necessary blood transfusions caused her to lose several layers of skin. Her body was covered with hives and rashes.

On Christmas Day, less than two weeks after she was admitted to the hospital, Beverly was in crisis. Her white-cell count had dropped severely, and her temperature rose to 105 degrees. She alternated between chills and convulsions, despite the attempts of the nurses to lower her temperature with alcohol baths. Finally the doctor came in. "We talked about this the first day," he said. "Penicillin might kill you, but I think it's the only thing we can do now. I'm going to ask you to sign this permission slip."

Slowly and painfully, Beverly signed it.

"I'm going to give you just a little," he said, "and wait fifteen minutes. If everything's okay, we'll try a little more." It was a terrifying experience—like playing Russian roulette—but Beverly's body tolerated the penicillin, and she escaped death that Christmas afternoon.

By New Year's Day the pretty young woman who had entered the hospital was hardly recognizable. She had lost twenty pounds and all of her long, beautiful brown hair. Both physically and emotionally, she was suffering intensely. Every three or four days the vein in her arm would collapse, and the IV would have to be moved to a new location.

But often it seemed to Beverly that her emotional pain was the harder to deal with. The nights were especially bad. "I was so lonely I thought I'd die from it," she says softly. "Lying there in bed, unable to sleep, I would fill up with doubt. Sometimes I could convince myself that I had as much chance as anybody of getting through this ordeal, and I'd feel a surge of strength. But then I would start to doubt my strength, and even my faith, and I'd feel totally defeated. Sometimes I cried all night. Other times I actually screamed."

Alone in her room, isolated from the rest of the hospital, Beverly spoke to God often. "At first I asked, 'Why me? This isn't fair! What have I done to deserve this?' Then I prayed for healing. Once I *demanded* that He heal me, but I knew that wasn't right. So I begged Him for healing, for the kids' sake and for Joe's sake. And I begged for some relief and peace. And there were times I was in so much pain I couldn't form the words to speak to God any longer."

For Beverly, wife of a minister, the illness was a turning point in her faith and understanding. Although she questioned God, ultimately her deep religious conviction moved her to an acceptance of her condition. "Finally I prayed, 'God, I love You, and I can't take this pain anymore. If You'll just hold my hand a little bit tighter, I know I can get through this.' And I did."

Beverly also turned to the Bible, looking for texts that

might help her understand. It was the Book of Job, with its examination of human suffering, that helped her most. She explains, "This is where Satan goes to God and says, 'I want to test your faithful servant Job. Look how good you've been to him, God. He's got everything. He's never had a test. How do you know he loves you?'

"So God says, 'He loves me.'

"But Satan says, 'I want him. Let me test him.'

"Then God spoke. 'All right. You can do anything you want with him, but you can't take his life. His life is mine.'

"When I studied that, it came to me that God was saying the same thing to me. I don't mean that I believe He said, 'I'm going to give Beverly Hall acute leukemia so she can prove herself.' I just feel that He had to allow evil forces in the world so we have something to compare the good against, and I was a random victim. But what I got out of Job was that I realized whatever might happen to me, God would see me through. My life is His. Nobody and no disease can take my life until God has decided that's the day. When I realized that, I didn't have anything to fret about anymore. I was able to accept the fact that I had leukemia, because I also had a loving God who would give me the everyday strength to go through whatever I must.

"I realized, down deep, 'I *can* do anything, not by myself, but through Christ.' So then I could accept it and have peace of mind. That peace of mind kept me going, and it's still what keeps me going every day."

Beverly's faith was a powerful antidote to her fear and despair. Once she recovered from her near-fatal crisis on Christmas Day, she asked Joe to bring her a hymnal. From then on, whenever she felt that depression was getting the best of her, she picked up the hymnal and began singing. "Whatever the emotion I felt at that moment, I could sing," she says. "And if I could just keep singing, I could keep from crying."

The support of family, friends, hospital staff, and even people she had never met was a great source of strength. Beverly's blue eyes brighten when she talks about it. "I had whole churches praying for me, people who had never seen me. Catholic friends sent me holy water, and Pentecostal friends wanted to come in and anoint me with oil so I would be healed. And I got so many cards! I still have what must be thousands of letters and get-well cards. It's lovely. It still does wonders for my spirits when I get a funny card, or a note in the mail from somebody who says, 'I'm thinking about you today.' Anything—knowing that people care is what really counts."

One of the most helpful presents Beverly received was a tape recorder, given by a group of friends. With this, she could record letters to people, as well as listen to their taped messages over and over. She also listened to religious music on the cassette player, and found great inspiration in it. "John Montgomery's *Joy Comes in the Morning* and John Shillington's *Sheltered in the Arms of God* were especially comforting to me."

The telephone by Beverly's bed was very important. Joe points out with a faint smile that she ran up some astronomical long-distance phone bills.

"It was good for me to talk to people in the outside world," she explains. "It's important to keep in touch. It's also important to keep occupied. I watched very little television, although I had a TV in my room. When it came down to it, I preferred to look at the nice things people had sent, the cards, little things everywhere, small figurines, a candle, a dried flower arrangement. They really made that hospital room beautiful."

Although Beverly had never thought of herself as a creative person, she began latch-hooking rugs and working with ceramics while in the hospital. She would sand pots, which Joe then took to a shop to be fired. When he brought them back, she would paint them. "I felt proud when the doctors and nurses came to my room to see them," she says. "To keep occupied and go on living, that's the important thing. You've got to realize that as long as you're alive, you must do something with your life."

While Beverly struggled to keep herself active, Joe had to learn to fit many new responsibilities into an already busy life. During the fifteen years of their marriage, running the household had been Beverly's responsibility. Now everything landed squarely on Joe's shoulders. "It was a shock," he says with a deep laugh. "I suppose I used to have that macho concept that a man was the head of the household, and it was a woman's duty to clean and care for the children. Traditional male thinking. Well, all of that vanished," he says with a snap of his fingers, "when Bev became sick. The carpets needed vacuuming and there was nobody to do it but me. And somebody had to get up at 6:30 in the morning to cook breakfast for the kids and get them off to school—and that somebody was me.

"I did the whole bit," he says, with satisfaction. "I found myself washing clothes, ironing clothes, taking Johnny to swimming lessons, and Krista to cheerleader practice, and Joe to football practice. Making dinner—the whole bit. I developed a routine. On Friday morning, when everyone was gone, I'd be in my underwear doing the major housecleaning. I'd take all the furniture out of a room, vacuum it, and move everything back. Then I'd do the next room, until the whole house was done.

"A man's got to be willing to make a lot of changes when his wife is severely ill," Joe says. "Believe me, his life is going to be radically different than it was. Don't think you're above getting down on your hands and knees to clean the commode. I've done it."

With the new burdens, Joe also had to make some professional adjustments. Shortly after Beverly first entered the hospital, he explained the situation to the leaders of his church.

"Now, I can take a leave of absence," he said, "or you people can share some of my responsibilities with me." The laymen gladly agreed to help him out. In addition, Joe asked several dedicated members of the congregation to prepare sermons and be on call, in case he should have to be at the hospital on a Sunday morning. "My congregation has been wonderful," he says. "They've helped me in every way I asked."

Even though relieved of some of his ministerial responsibilities, Joe still found it difficult to fit everything in—especially personal time when he could be alone and gather his own resources. He soon learned that he could not spend every free moment in Beverly's hospital room. "The spouse who's not sick has to retain his or her own identity," he says. "It hurts me to think of Bev alone in her hospital room, bored to tears. When she's been hospitalized, I've spent a great deal of time with her. But I can't be there all the time. The reality is that *she* is the one in the hospital. She is the one who has leukemia. I don't. The children don't. They have to be taken care of and educated; they have to grow. So I have many responsibilities to them, and I also have a responsibility to myself. It's not good for me or anyone to try to take someone's disease and carry part of it—and of course it's something I can't do, anyway. The sad fact is, I can't experience what she's experiencing. I have to continue with my own life.

"If Bev were to die," he says more slowly, "a major part of me would die along with her. But I can't allow all of me to die. I can't become totally engrossed with grief. If I did, all hell would break loose with my kids, my profession, everything."

Beverly points out that she and Joe have arrived at a common understanding of this problem slowly, and only after many discussions and disagreements. "There have been times when I needed him to love and reassure me," she says, "and he wasn't there. One of the worst fights we ever had was over a Saturday afternoon when he went out to play golf. I really got upset. Dr. Leichtman happened to come in when I was crying, and asked me what the problem was.

"I told him, 'I'm angry with Joe. He's out playing golf and I need him here with me.'

"Dr. Leichtman said to me, 'You've got to give him his space.'

"In time I realized that was good advice. Joe had to get away and unwind now and then. The poor guy had almost no time by himself, and he just needed to get out on the golf course alone that afternoon and enjoy the outdoors. It was therapy for him."

Both Beverly and Joe have had to confront personal guilt during her illness. For Joe, overcoming guilt meant learning to respect his need for relaxation and personal time. Beverly's guilt stemmed from her realization of what Joe and the children had to cope with because of her illness. "I'm very fortunate, though," she says. "When I feel really bad I can just have a good cry, and in an hour I'm over it. Joe doesn't let his emotions out that easily."

From the beginning, the young couple shared another major concern: medical expenses. When Beverly first entered the hospital, neither she nor Joe knew whether the family's group insurance would cover her expenses, which might run as much as $100,000 that first year. Since Beverly was starting a new job, her new employer's policy did not cover her yet.

Sitting on her bed at night, in isolation, Beverly prayed, "Please don't let us go bankrupt." Her prayer was answered, she believes, and in a way she never expected. Her former employer had not yet canceled her insurance; she was still covered, and had the right to convert to an individual policy. She did, and her medical expenses were covered by two policies—Joe's group insurance, and hers.

As a result, not only were Beverly's medical bills paid, but to their amazement, the Halls received money from the second insurance company over and above what they needed to pay the bills. Hardly able to believe this windfall was real, Joe called the Michigan Department of Insurance and explained the situation. He wanted to make sure that he was entitled to the double coverage. He was delighted to be told, "You have paid extra premiums for the right to collect from two insurers for the same loss; therefore you are entitled to collect from both of them."

Most of the extra insurance money is now carefully invested, and will provide security for the future and pay for the education of the Halls' children. "And as it turned out," Joe says, "we've also been able to give our children things they would not have had otherwise."

In the third month of Beverly's hospitalization Dr. Leichtman pushed her to consider a life-and-death decision. Would she gamble her life on a bone marrow transplant? The donor must be a sibling of the leukemia patient; because of the severity of Beverly's leukemia, the chromosome match with the donor would have to be perfect. The decision to have the transplant was a grave one, since it carried with it a high risk. It would mean that Beverly would again be put in isolation, and would be given massive chemotherapy to eradicate all her own bone marrow. Then, while she was maintained on life-support systems, the bone marrow from the donor would be transplanted. There was a real risk that Beverly might die during this procedure.

If the transplant worked, the doctor explained, Beverly would be cured of her acute leukemia, and eventually be able to live a normal life again. The odds were against her surviving the operation, however. On the other hand, without the transplant she could die in a short time. Only Beverly and Joe could decide whether the risk was worth taking.

"It was a question of whether or not I wanted to go for it and gamble on winning," Beverly says with a thoughtful expression. "If I did, I'd be going for broke. I could choose instead to have those last few months with my husband and children. I thought and prayed about it, and finally decided against the operation. There were so many things I'd never gotten around to sharing with my children, so many things to talk to them about, that I wanted to go home and be with them."

Dr. Leichtman respected Beverly's decision, and he added that she herself should feel comfortable with her choice from then on. "Try not to second-guess yourself," he said.

In April 1980, Beverly was released from the hospital. During the next two months she enjoyed her time with Joe and the children. She received a monthly "maintenance treatment" of chemotherapy injections at the doctor's office. In July, however, she was back in the hospital with a blood infection.

"I was furious about it!" she exclaims. "Somehow I'd been under the impression that I'd never have to be in a hospital again. I thought I'd live the remainder of my short life at home, spending time with the kids, doing everything I wanted to do. I thought perhaps we'd go on a trip. And I'd been feeling fairly good—it was great being out of the hospital. But now I was back in! It wasn't what I'd bargained for!" Feeling cheated, Beverly thought, "I've gone through so much. Why can't I have my last months without being sick in the hospital?"

After only a week, however, she was released and returned home to her family. But one month later she was back in the hospital for another week, this time to have an internal rectal fistula removed, which had resulted from the chemotherapy. Then, in September, when Beverly was in Dr. Leichtman's office for her monthly maintenance treatment, he told her she would have to enter the hospital again for a "consolidation treatment." This, he explained, would help her stay in remission.

Beverly was so angry she burst into tears. The doctor assured her it was necessary, but she envisioned an endless succession of hospitalizations.

"Isn't there *anything* I can do besides spend the rest of my life in the hospital?" she pleaded.

Dr. Leichtman looked at her and said, "You can still have a bone marrow transplant. That's your only option, Beverly. Otherwise, this is it."

Beverly squared her shoulders and asked him what her chances were now without the transplant. Of adults over thirty with her disease, he explained, 50 percent died between the tenth and fourteenth months. Beverly thought, "I'm now in my eighth month. The odds are stacking up against me." Suddenly she wanted to fight with everything she had.

At home that evening she talked with Joe about it, and then prayed. "I said to God, 'Okay, Lord, I'm just going to leave it in Your hands. You told Satan he could not take Job's life, and I know you won't let this disease take mine. I'm going to live every day you intend me to live—whether I have this bone marrow transplant or not.'" Beverly also thought deeply on what the transplant would mean for their family life if it were successful. "It would be so much easier without all the anxiety we'd had, without all the fretting. It would give us a definite answer. Either life would be victoriously sweet and happy for my family, or they'd be able to set about rebuilding their lives without me. So I called Dr. Leichtman to say I wanted to do it."

The doctor told Beverly he wanted her to take a full week to be certain of her decision; she agreed. But the next day she felt so positive that she called his office and insisted that she would not be changing her mind.

Now that the decision was made, Beverly was riding on a wave of optimism and anticipation. Arrangements were completed to test the blood samples from her brothers and sisters. She hoped that her brother in Seattle would be the donor, since he lived near a leading hospital where the transplant could be done. Finally the results of the tests came in, and they were devastating. Her chromosomes did not match those of any of her four siblings. The bone marrow transplant was impossible.

Terribly disappointed, Beverly cried when she got the news. But she realized she would have to put it behind her. She had missed last Christmas, and in fact had nearly died on Christmas Day. This year she would have Christmas at home. She absorbed herself in planning for the holidays, and began to live again. In time she has become more reconciled to her illness. For example, she no longer panics when she experiences pain. "I came to really understand my blessings," she says softly. "I've got a wonderful family and an excellent doctor and so many friends—I've got a lot going for me. I keep busy now, and I even dream about things I want to do in the future. Now I don't go around thinking I'm going to die any day."

Leukemia has changed Beverly in more visible ways, too. In her first, crucial bout with the illness she lost twenty pounds and two dress sizes and all of her hair. She has gained forty-six pounds since then and "several dress sizes—I won't say how many." Her hair that has regrown is thin and brittle, and she wears it in a short pixie style. "It was very traumatic to lose my hair," she admits. "It just fell out in handfuls when I was first in the hospital; I kept finding it on my bed. Of course, I was having a hard time just then, and losing my hair made me feel like I'd been stripped. My hair was the one thing that made me feel a little bit pretty, and I thought, 'Now I'll never be pretty again.'"

At first, embarrassed, Beverly covered her head with a scarf, so that the nurses and doctors who entered her room wouldn't see her baldness. Later, Joe brought her a wig. But both the scarf and the wig were uncomfortable, since the nerve endings in her head were sensitive. In the hospital and later at home, she tended less and less to cover her head. "It was funny," she says with a smile. "I'd go around the house baldheaded, but if somebody came to the door, I'd start frantically running around looking for my wig."

Beverly decided not to hide her hair loss from the children, since it was just another facet of her illness. Johnny, her youngest son, quickly brought the issue to the surface when he visited her in her hospital room. He looked with awe at her uncovered head, his eyes large, and blurted out, "Hey, Mom, you look like a monster!" While Beverly initially was hurt by this, Joe encouraged her to laugh about the incident. As a result, Johnny became so accepting of his mother's baldness that he came home one day with a request that she come to school with him the next morning for Show and Tell, so his classmates could see her. "I refrained from that," Beverly says dryly.

As her hair slowly grew back in, Beverly grew less self-conscious. Eventually, rather than endure the discomfort of the wig, she even did her grocery shopping without covering her head. "There were a few people who stared," she admits, "but I'd just smile at them. Really, most people paid no attention to my hair style. But I had learned to accept myself, and that's what's important."

By February 1982 Beverly felt good enough to fly to San Antonio, Texas, to visit her sixty-one-year-old father, who was being treated in a clinic for terminal lung cancer. His cancer was inoperable, and Beverly wanted to spend time with him while she had a chance. Her visit was extremely important to him. He proudly introduced her to everyone: "This is my daughter, Beverly. She's had leukemia for over a year, but look at her now!"

Unfortunately, while she was in San Antonio, Beverly picked up a viral blood infection, and began running a high temperature. She flew back to Detroit, where Joe picked her up at the airport and rushed her to Providence Hospital. There she was again a patient, this time for seventeen days.

During her remission, Beverly has been hospitalized more frequently than she ever expected. While she dislikes being away from the family, she has grown to accept this as a periodic necessity. In the same way, she has learned to accept the pain she once thought she could not endure. Perhaps the worst pain has come from injections directly to her spine. These become necessary when she began to experience severe headaches. Dr. Leichtman concluded that the chemotherapy, administered through her bloodstream, was not effectively combating the leukemia cells that were likely to be in her spinal column. To reach these cells, he had to give her injections directly into the spine, by way of a hole drilled between the lower vertebrae.

The injections at this site caused scar tissue to build up over time, making it increasingly difficult to insert the needle in the right spot. The pain was such that Joe stood beside his wife during the injections, holding her hand and comforting her. "Sometimes the needle would slip and go right into her bone," he says with a wince. "She'd just grit her teeth and grip my hand until both our hands turned white. At first she'd scream, but now she doesn't anymore. And that's the same girl who used to panic at the thought of a simple shot. She's come a long way."

In many ways, Beverly feels her relationships have become deeper and more satisfying. "First," she says, "my relationship with God is so much more solid now. I often think of Psalm 17, where God tells David to test Him, and He will show He is God. I don't know of a more shattering crisis I could ever encounter than this, and God brought me through it. I don't think I could ever doubt Him again. The second thing is my family. I realize now just how beautiful my husband and children are. They're everything I need. Material things have a lower priority with me than they once did; they're nice, but knowing that somebody loves you and cares for you is far more meaningful. And it's wonderful to have a chance to return their love. We're much closer now. This illness has led me to see how much the love of my family means to me."

Her illness has also led Beverly to appreciate little things far more than she once did. She remembers one autumn Sunday afternoon when she had a pass from the hospital, and spent the day at home. While Joe and the boys watched a football game on television, she and her daughter took a walk around the block. "I got so much joy out of that," she says, "just hearing the trees rustle in the wind and the leaves crackle under my feet, and feeling the wind in my hair. I don't remember ever enjoying that when my hair was shoulder-length. Now it was only an inch long, and it felt so nice in the breeze. I mentioned that later to Dr. Leichtman, and he understood. He just smiled and said, 'I know.'"

Although Beverly had yet to receive a clean bill of health, she felt confident enough to relocate to Tucson, Arizona, where her husband has a new congregation, and she plans to go back to college and earn a degree. As an experienced patient, she has definite ideas on how a hospital should operate, and would like to go into hospital administration.

According to the latest medical reports, Beverly's debilitation is now more related to chemotherapy than to her leukemia. Joe cautiously says that he believes her body will naturally rebuild itself once she is off chemotherapy. Beverly reminds him that she may need more chemotherapy at any time.

Beverly still has leukemia, and both she and Joe are aware of the fact that no one can predict how long she will live. "Regardless of that she's still a survivor," Joe says. "What you do with your life, the quality of your life, that's what it's all about. And in this respect, Bev is a survivor."

Beverly has come a long way; according to Dr. Leichtman, she has already lived longer than any patient in her age group, with her type of leukemia, that he has ever treated. It has been a difficult time for her. In the first thirty months of her illness she spent over three hundred days in the hospital. She knows that she faces the possibility of a recurrence at any time. "But I'm still alive and fighting," she says optimistically. "And life has so much meaning to me now."

8

RENA TARBET

In a speech to eight thousand women at a recent Mary Kay Cosmetics convention in Dallas, the company's number one sales director said, "I learned some valuable lessons this year, and I'd like to share a few of them with you. I learned that we must live one day at a time; we plan for tomorrow, but we must live for today. I have learned that it isn't really what happens to us that matters, but how we respond to what happens. And I've learned that life doesn't have to be easy to be a pleasure. . . ."

When Rena Tarbet concluded her short speech, she received a standing ovation. There wasn't a dry eye in the house—and for good reason. Her audience knew of her struggle with cancer and her fierce determination not to be defeated by it.

Rena's strong faith, high spirits, and unyielding determination have led her to the top of Mary Kay Cosmetics, an international company with 200,000 sales consultants. On center stage at the convention, she looks magnificent. At 5 feet 5 inches and 120 pounds she is slender, with a beautiful complexion and curly blond hair. Her mink stole and gold jewelry are symbols of success to the women in the audience, who know they are hard-won awards for her achievements in sales management. Her talk is delivered with the poise and emphasis of the seasoned speaker she is.

Rena cannot talk long without referring to her career. In 1967, when she joined the cosmetics firm, Rena, her husband, Eddie, and their three children had just moved to Fort Worth. Rena's ambition when she became a beauty consultant was to augment the family's monthly income of $300 with perhaps $30 a week, to help pay the bills.

To her surprise, Rena found she could not only sell, she could inspire other women to sell, too. Before long she was heading her own sales organization. By 1975, Rena was earning so much that Eddie was able to quit his job, where he was unhappy, and find more fulfilling work, even though it brought in less money. At thirty-two, Rena had found her niche, and "things were going great. I had the best of two worlds—a happy, healthy family, and a marvelous career.

"That was the year I discovered a lump in my left breast. *Crunch.*"

Rena's gynecologist congratulated her for having done regular self-examinations, and told her she had nothing to worry about. He set up an appointment for the following day with a surgeon who would do a mammogram and needle biopsy. Both tests came back negative. In high spirits, Rena entered the hospital for an overnight stay, preparatory to having the lump removed in the morning. She was so unconcerned about the surgery that she hadn't even called any friends; nobody but Eddie even knew about the surgery. It was "just no big deal."

Rena and the doctors were wrong. The pathology report sent back to the operating room proved that the tumor was malignant. The malignancy was such a surprise that the doctors had not even asked Rena to sign standard release papers giving permission for radical surgery if necessary. Since Rena was still under anesthetic, the surgeon now asked Eddie to sign the release, explaining that he believed a radical mastectomy was essential. Without hesitation, Eddie signed the paper, sure that Rena would make the same decision.

When Rena awoke in the recovery room, she was surprised to find her husband, two of her closest friends, and the surgeon at her bedside. As she fought drowsiness, she heard the surgeon speaking. "I'm very sorry, we had to take it all." She drifted in and out of consciousness, hearing those words. "We had to take it all."

Once she was fully awake and understood what had happened, Rena was shocked by the news. For two days she felt depressed, a period of time she does not like to talk about. "Depression is not part of my self-image. Then I thought, 'Big deal,' and I snapped right back. They told me they got it all and everything was going to be fine. So I decided I could get along just as well as ever. Life goes on."

Eddie, whom Rena describes as a very calm man and an eternal optimist, has a very strong faith in God. "He has never seemed shaken by my cancer. From the moment I woke up after surgery, he's told me, 'Don't worry, honey, everything will be all right.' No matter what has happened, he's always told me that. 'Hey, everything will be all right.'"

Forced to remain in the hospital for nearly two weeks, Rena soon decided she wouldn't let that slow her down. By the end of the week she had set up shop in her hospital room and was busily working with her sales organization via telephone, Rolodex and IBM sheets spread out all over the bed. One intern who entered her room to find her like this was taken aback.

"Lady," he said, "what in the world is going *on?*"

"I'm taking care of my business."

"You're awfully hyper. What are you on?"

"I'm not on anything."

"Hold out your hand."

Rena did. "Well, it's not shaking," the intern said.

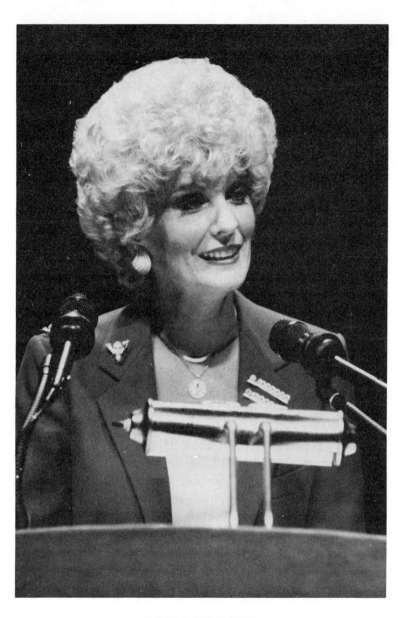

RENA TARBET

"I told you I wasn't on anything," she said. "It's sheer enthusiasm."

Rena was undoubtedly a happening in the Fort Worth hospital. Not only was her room an office, but it held so many gift plants and flowers it looked like a florist shop. Dozens of friends and associates made their way through the greenery, including her hairdresser. "Let me tell you," Rena says, "once I adjusted to the mastectomy, I didn't slow down at all. Not at *all*."

Determined to keep going, Rena kept a business commitment three days after her release from the hospital—and she did it with as much vitality as ever. "I was off and running!" she says happily. "It was as if I'd never had cancer. My doctor recommended no follow-up treatment, and I soon felt as energetic as ever."

Rena had thought of reconstructive surgery while still hospitalized, and she included it on her list of questions for the doctor. "In my sales career," she explains, "I learned to always make up a list of the most important things to do every day, and I just naturally made a list of important questions for my doctor, too. One of them was about reconstruction, and he immediately said he was against it. But I'd think about it, and it would go back on that list, and I'd ask him again.

"Every time I'd ask him about it, he'd say, 'Rena, you're inviting trouble. That's like having lung cancer and then going back to smoking. I'm absolutely against it.'"

"I simply forgot I'd even had cancer. I was feeling perfectly healthy. Life was just great."

By November 1979, four years had passed since Rena's mastectomy. One day she realized that she had never lost her desire to have reconstructive surgery. A fashion-conscious woman, she wanted more freedom in choosing her clothes. "If I had reconstruction, I'd be able to wear things like spaghetti-strap dresses, pretty lingerie, and swim suits that I shied away from. And I wouldn't have to worry about a prosthesis." She made an appointment with a highly recommended plastic surgeon in San Antonio.

The last thing she expected was for the plastic surgeon to find a suspicious area in her right breast. He did. The results of the tests he ordered, along with Rena's history of breast cancer, led him to suggest a modified mastectomy on her right breast, to be performed at the same time as the reconstruction of her left breast.

In comparison to her radical mastectomy, the modified operation didn't seem serious. Instead of being upset, Rena focused on the fact that by sheer good luck the tumor had been found at a very early stage.

The double operation went smoothly, although the reconstruction was only partially completed with the first surgery. Two more operations were required over the next several months. "He had to build up my breast from nothing," Rena explains, "and he didn't have much to start with because so much tissue had been removed when they did the radical. Then it was a matter of taking a tuck in the skin here or there, and changing the size of the implants again and again so everything was balanced."

Rena had no complaints about the three surgeries, for the results were worth the trouble. Since then she has addressed a number of nursing classes on this subject, and talked to many women individually. "I always tell them how much more confident my reconstruction made me feel," she says. "It boosted my self-image—it just did so much for me. I feel more feminine and free. I've seen women who were decimated by the loss of a breast. They lost their sex drive; they felt mutilated and ugly. Reconstruction can do wonders for women who feel that way. I was such a confident person to begin with, and it helped me. Imagine what it can do for a woman

who isn't self-confident! So when people ask me what I think
of reconstruction surgery, I tell them that I personally recommend it very highly."

Again, Rena felt she had left cancer behind her. The surgeon had assured her that all cancerous cells had been removed, and follow-up treatment was unnecessary.

The only shadow on her successful life was an on-again,
off-again pain in her chest that began in the spring of 1980. It
was a definite pain, sometimes severe, but she assumed it
came from adhesions, since she'd had three operations within
the past year. Just when she began to wonder about the pain,
it would disappear, only to return a day or two later.

The summer passed, and although she tried to ignore it, the
pain did not disappear. Finally, one autumn day, the pain
was so severe Rena could hardly get out of bed. She went to
see the plastic surgeon, expecting him to confirm that the
problem was caused by adhesions.

That was not his diagnosis. Instead he told her to check into
a hospital.

The long day of testing seemed endless, and even Rena was
having difficulty feeling positive about it. "I was getting to be
an experienced patient," she says, "and I was familiar with
certain procedures. So when they would come up and say,
'We want to run this test again, Mrs. Tarbet,' I had suspicions.
They did several reruns, and they started to approach me
with that hush-hush way they have. It was that, more than
anything, that made me suspect what was coming."

Although she was braced for bad news, Rena did not expect to receive it the way she did. At the end of the day she
was approached by a radiologist she had never met, who said,
"Lady, I do not know how you're standing up and walking
around."

"I just have a lot of stamina."

"You must," he said grimly. "Your sternum is totally disintegrated by cancer. It looks like a piece of Swiss cheese."

As he talked on, Rena was swept by a wave of cold fear. She had come alone for the tests, and had no one to turn to. She had never been so shocked and frightened in her life.

Rena tries to see the very best in other people; however, this man tested her limits. "He had no compassion," she says. "He knew I was alone, and he should have called in a social worker or a counselor or called for my husband. It was just plain cruel to blurt it out like that. He was cruel."

As soon as she could, Rena called Eddie at work. Unwilling to explain on the phone, she told him, "I'm at the hospital. Can you go home now? I'll meet you there."

Eddie asked no questions. "I'll leave right away."

Rena was crying when Eddie came in. "I've got cancer again." She began to sob. "It's terrible. Every time I get up, I'm knocked down again. I'm the one who tells everybody that the mark of a champion is to get up when you're knocked down, but every time I get up I get knocked back down. Eddie, I feel defeated this time."

"Look at it this way," Eddie responded. "You had cancer once—you got better. You had cancer a second time—you got better. Now you have cancer a third time. Sure, it's serious. But it's time to get better again, now, not time to despair. Honey, don't worry. We'll do whatever we need to do."

On the advice of a friend who was a physician, Rena sought a second opinion at M. D. Anderson Hospital in Houston. Extensive testing confirmed the original diagnosis: she had cancer of the bone, originating in the sternum. It was no comfort to be told that this metastasis was not uncommon for the type of breast cancer she'd had.

For the first time Rena was put on a chemotherapy program. Every three weeks she went to Anderson, where she was first given intravenous chemotherapy for sixty to ninety minutes. Then a portable pump was hooked into a catheter below her collarbone. For the next four days, around the clock, Rena received chemotherapy through the catheter, one drop at a time.

The detailed instructions on how to care for the pump and replace the small vials of medicine were challenging. And Rena rather enjoyed another challenge—trying to get through the procedures at Anderson in one day and be back home that evening. It was a long day. She caught the first plane out of Fort Worth at 7:00 in the morning, and did not usually get home until about 11:00 at night. "But it was better than staying overnight and losing so much time!" she says. "I made a game out of it. I'd book five different flights under different names, so I'd be guaranteed a seat."

On the flight back, Rena looked like any other tired business person at the end of the day. The small pump which hung down from her neck was easily concealed by a jacket or sweater. She often talked to other passengers, and no one ever knew that at that moment she was receiving chemotherapy. Rena herself felt very positive about the process. Rather than lying in a chemotherapy ward, she was on her way home, receiving therapy but independent. At the end of the four days she would unhook the pump and send it back to the hospital. "I could go home and go about my business there, although I will admit I didn't feel too great, and I pretty much stayed at home during those four days."

Rena found that during the time her chemotherapy was being administered, she felt very weak, and was often nauseated. Reluctantly, she decided she could not sell or speak publicly during those days, since "it's difficult to feel enthusiastic when you're not feeling good, and enthusiasm is vital in sales."

For all her problems during the nine-month chemotherapy program, Rena continued to set national sales records in Mary Kay Cosmetics. Aside from her rare down days, she usually managed to keep her determination.

"I was at the hospital one day, and I had an important meeting to conduct the following morning," she says, "so I was determined to finish up that day. But toward the end of the afternoon, my doctor decided he had to have one more X ray. And when the nurse tried to arrange it, the X-ray department told her they were closing for the day, and it would have to wait till morning.

"I said, 'I have to be in Dallas in the morning. Let me talk to the doctor about this.' Well, I couldn't get in to see the doctor, so I waited until I caught him in the hall. And really quick, without pausing, I said to him, "Is there any reason why you couldn't call the X-ray department and ask them to see just one more patient?' Well, beginning with 'Is there any reason why' is a sales technique I've learned. Most of the time when you put a question that way, people can't really think of any reason why they can't do what you ask.

"So I just kept talking to him, explaining at ninety miles an hour: 'I-have-to-be-home-tomorrow-for-a-very-important-appointment-I'm-giving-a-workshop. Couldn't-you-just-call-the-X-ray-department-and-get-them-to-do-just-one-more-X-ray?'

"He looked at me for a minute and broke out laughing. Then he picked up the phone and called the X-ray department. The wonderful thing was that *he* used my technique on *them*. He started right out asking them, 'Is there any reason why you couldn't do just one more X ray this afternoon?' Well, it worked, and I got my X ray, and got out of there, and caught the late plane, and I did my workshop the next day!"

Because of her positive attitude, Rena was strikingly different in appearance from most of the other patients at the hospital. It bothered her to see them. "So many of them looked like they had lost hope," she says. "The women didn't bother to wear makeup anymore; some of them never even wore their wigs. I just couldn't do that. The doctors notice these things, too. One of them said to me, 'Rena, for so many patients cancer becomes a full-time project, and their whole life centers around it. But you're working the cancer around other things in your life. They're dying with cancer. *You're living with it.*"

Like many cancer patients, Rena also had to live with the loss of her hair. When she began chemotherapy, she was warned that this might happen, and purchased several wigs in preparation. Her hair did begin to come out in clumps, each time she combed it or scratched her head. In March 1981, fourteen days after her first chemotherapy treatment, Rena was scheduled to go on a trip to Spain, a special award for the top ten Mary Kay performers. As the time grew nearer and her hair grew patchier, she got more and more aggravated with the process. Finally, on the night before the trip, she stood in front of the bathroom mirror "and picked the hair out. It was so loose, there was nothing to it, and I just plucked at it like you'd pluck a chicken until it was gone. My daughter Kim, who was sixteen at the time, sat there and watched me, and when I was through she put her arms around me and said, 'I love you, Mama.'"

The next morning Rena left for Spain. She was number one in the company that year—"but I sure didn't feel like it!" True, with her well-styled wig and beautiful clothes, she looked as attractive as ever. "But I didn't feel very pretty," she says, momentarily downcast at the memory. "*I* knew it was a wig. Well, I learned a long time ago that sometimes you have to 'fake it to make it,' and act enthusiastic when you don't feel that way. I was determined to enjoy that trip, and the last thing I needed was people saying, 'God love her, she has cancer.' I don't need sympathy. I was *not* going to let that cancer interfere with my enjoyment of that trip, and it didn't. I had a terrific time in Spain."

Like some cancer patients, Rena has gained a great deal of strength and courage from support persons outside her immediate family. Many patients find it can be difficult to communicate such feelings as fear and discouragement to family members—even to their spouses. Often a husband or wife is so emotionally involved that the patient's sickness is his or her own sickness, too. In addition, psychologists who work with cancer patients caution against the patient leaning too heavily on any one person. Even the most loving husband or wife may eventually be overwhelmed or become unavailable. Through her work, Rena has developed a broad support system which includes some "special friends." One such support person is Paul Van Dyke, a company sales executive who became a personal friend over the years.

To many Mary Kay people, Rena seems to be a super-woman, and their affection for her is tinged with a kind of awe. "But I'm not always up," Rena explains, "and there are times when I feel as lonely and frightened as anyone. I need someone who can accept the fact that I'm not superhuman, someone I can cry my heart out to. Paul's that person.

"At times he can help me in ways Eddie can't—just as Eddie sometimes helps me at times when I wouldn't dream of calling Paul. All of my friends have something to offer, each according to who they are. I'm just lucky to have so many good friends."

Rena believes much of her strength comes from her faith in God. Instead of seeing cancer as a meaningless intrusion in her life, she believes it is part of God's design. "In a sense, I see my life like the underside of a weaving. To me it may look like an ugly pattern with broken thread and knots, but God is above, looking at the beautiful design." She also believes that she has a purpose in life. Today, almost all of the May Kay beauty consultants know of her history with cancer and her courage. Her inspiring example to them now goes far beyond sales motivation. One consultant, Linda Snyder of Schenectady, New York, suffered a severed spinal cord in an automobile accident in mid-1982. Now paralyzed from the waist down, Linda keeps Rena's photograph on her dresser for inspiration. "You see," Rena says, "God has been able to use me to touch the lives of thousands of women. I feel there are a lot more women out there for me to reach, and that He needs me more down here than up there. That's why I believe I will be given more time on this earth."

Like every cancer patient, Rena has to deal with the uncertainty of her future. She firmly believes that the best way to do this is to set long-term goals and work toward them. "Life doesn't give anybody guarantees," she says. "We all have to take it one day at a time. And there's no use worrying about what happens to you—it's how you respond to it that matters."

The Tarbet family has learned to accept Rena's cancer with the same good grace. From the beginning, Rena and Eddie have kept the children informed of what was happening to her. Rena says, "It's almost as though we have six members in our family—Eddie, me, the three children, and then there's Cancer. But it's no big deal, we've learned to live with it. The kids have adjusted very well. For example, sometimes I don't wear a wig around the house. So the kids learned that if they brought a friend home after school, as soon as they hit the door they should holler out, 'Hey, Mom, Steve's with me.' That way if I'm not presentable I can put myself together."

Rena has been concerned about developing independence in the children. "If I'm not here for my family, they must adjust and go on. I've worked hard to make sure that if I'm not around, my children won't become emotional cripples. I know they'll miss me, but I want them to be able to adjust. I've taught them to be secure within themselves, and I praise them constantly to build their self-confidence. I've taught them that they don't need me or anyone else in order to get what they want out of life."

Whatever else, Rena hopes her children know how to persevere. A favorite saying of hers is, "Never give in, never give up, and never give out." She preaches this determination both to her children and to the thousands of women in her sales organization, and she practices it herself. "Whether it's my business or my struggle with cancer, I'm always in there fighting," she says. "And I always have an alternative plan, so I'm never knocked out by defeat. The one thing I don't do is feel sorry for myself and have a pity party."

After several months, Rena's chemotherapy at Anderson was discontinued because her body was no longer responding positively to the drugs. Next she received cobalt treatments for twenty consecutive days at Moncrief Radiation Center in Fort Worth. This local hospital was more convenient, so Rena interrupted her schedule only to run in each afternoon for a treatment. "Cobalt never slowed me down," she says. "I saw patients throw up even before the treatments, before a needle hit their vein or the radiation light turned on. I believe so much of being sick is up here, in the mind."

In November of 1981 Rena finished the cobalt treatments. Now the plan called for a two-week rest, followed by renewed chemotherapy. During this time, a friend urged Rena to visit a nutritionist, "just to hear what he has to say."

"Why not?" Rena said. "What have I got to lose?"

The nutritionist reviewed Rena's medical history and gave her an entirely different recommendation on treatment. "Let me say this up front," he began. "You've cut your chances of survival in half by having chemotherapy and cobalt. I wish I could have gotten to you before that." While Rena sat dumbfounded, he went on, "I can't make you any long-term guarantees, but I will say you will live longer on my nutrition program than you will on conventional therapy methods."

"What?"

"You need to take a bold step. There comes a time when you have to make your own decisions. No matter what the doctors tell you, it's you, the patient, who has to decide. It's your body; you've got to do right by it."

Rena was too shaken to make a decision. She told the nutritionist she would talk to him again the next day.

One hour later Rena had an appointment with her oncologist. She told him she was thinking of leaving standard therapy to work with the nutritionist. As she expected, the oncologist firmly believed chemotherapy was necessary. He told her, "Rena, you're a total fool if you don't continue on chemotherapy. Please, listen to what they told you at M. D. Anderson."

"Lord," Rena says, "*I* didn't know the answer! I was a layman, and I didn't know what to do." She drove home crying and praying for some kind of guidance.

When she walked in the house, the first thing she saw was her mail. The first letter she opened included an article on nutrition. Rena recognized the author's name, and went looking in the stack of books she hadn't gotten around to reading yet. As she thought, she had a book on nutrition by the same man. She sat the rest of the day reading the article and the book. Everything in them agreed with what the nutritionist had said. In her confusion, she interpreted the coincidence as an omen. She called the nutritionist and said, "I'll be there tomorrow!"

"Great," he said. "We'll shave your head and start the analysis."

Rena had only half an inch of hair—it had just started to grow back. She was dismayed to think she would now lose it all—but she was not put off.

From November 1981 through mid-March of the following year, Rena worked with the nutritionist, her only treatment consisting of a diet she describes as "high doses of vitamins, especially vitamin C, lots of supplements, fresh fruits and vegetables, whole grain cereals, loads of enzymes, and carrot juice."

The diet, however, did not rid Rena of her cancer. Her deteriorating health and lack of energy became evident to her long-time friend, Mary Kay Ash. Over the years, the business relationship between the two women had developed into an affectionate friendship. Mary Kay was then convalescing from a rare virus which had had her in and out of the hospital for several months. She called Rena from her hospital room in Wadley Institute of Molecular Medicine and asked her to come and visit.

"Well," Rena says, "I became a little suspicious, because it wasn't like Mary Kay to ask somebody to visit her in the hospital, but of course I told her I'd be right there."

When she arrived at Wadley, Rena found Mary Kay looking well, and the two women chatted for a while. In the course of their conversation, Mary Kay repeatedly praised her physician, Dr. Amanullah Khan. Before long, Dr. Khan stopped in while making his rounds—and stayed to talk. After a while, Rena became suspicious again, knowing that doctors didn't stay that long with any one patient while making their rounds. Then Mary Kay casually asked, "Rena, I've told Dr. Khan about you, but why don't you tell him. I'm sure you can explain your situation a lot better than I can."

At this point, Rena was sure Mary Kay had set up this meeting—but she was also sure it was motivated only by concern. She told the doctor her history. He expressed interest, and asked if she would sign releases so he could review her medical records.

"I consented," Rena remembers. "But I told him in no uncertain terms that I was convinced nutrition was the answer to my health problems, and I would never go back on chemotherapy. Then Mary Kay said to him, 'You cure my girl, and I'll finance your research.'"

Touched by Mary Kay's concern, Rena was nevertheless stubborn. "I told Dr. Khan, 'I'm a better salesperson than you are, and you've got a whale of a job to convince me I'm on the wrong track.'"

A few weeks later, in Dr. Khan's office, Rena was hit with

some very disturbing, and convincing, news. After reviewing her records, the doctor had asked her to come to Wadley for extensive tests. The results revealed three new tumors—in her skull, left shoulder, and lower back.

"We need to take immediate action," Dr. Khan told her. "You should be on chemotherapy."

In spite of the new tumors, Rena said her faith in nutrition had not swayed. But Dr. Khan explained that he believed in nutrition, too. He told her, "Nutrition *will* build up your immune system and serve as a detoxification program. But I do not believe in *only* nutrition or only radiation or only chemo. I believe in a combination of treatments. You need chemotherapy because chemotherapy kills cancer cells."

"It also kills good cells," Rena protested.

"Yes, it does—but it kills, and that's the most important thing. Nutrition isn't going to kill the cancer in the time we have to work with. You need chemotherapy now!"

Rena decided to take Dr. Khan's advice. Today she still takes vitamins, over sixty pills a day. In addition, she is back on a twenty-one-day cycle of chemotherapy, with one day of intravenous treatment, four days of oral medication, four days of no treatment, and seven days of interferon, an experimental drug which presently costs about $1,000 a shot to administer. Following the interferon shots, she has "five good days—days with no treatment. The effects of the interferon are relatively mild—a slight chill, some aches and a fever, sort of like the flu." During her first treatment, Dr. Khan kept Rena in the hospital for observation overnight. After that, she insisted she wanted to be at home, and she got her way.

While Rena seems to be responding to the new program, it is too soon to predict her future. In the meantime, she is still going ninety miles an hour. "The Good Lord, the doctors, and I are going to lick it! I've got cancer, but I didn't choose it, and I'm not going to dedicate my life to it. It's not going to take me over.

"That old saying, 'It doesn't matter if you win or lose, it's how you play the game,' that's a bunch of hooey! You play to win. You give it all you've got, every bit of yourself. And when the final whistle blows, if you don't come out on top, it's okay, because you know you gave it your best."

Rena pauses briefly and concludes, "I play to win. I *know* I'm going to beat it!"

9

JOAN HEGERMAN

At the April 1972 Shaklee Corporation sales convention in Wichita, Kansas, Joan Hegerman had a wonderful time—as usual. During the ten years she and Al had been distributors for the giant food supplement company, they had played a major role in building the Midwest market. Joan knew everybody, it seemed, and conventions were practically family reunions. Moreover, since the Hegermans headed a sizable sales organization, Joan was often approached for advice and asked to speak at meetings.

One night during the convention, Joan and her roommate were kept awake by the rustling sounds of a small mouse somewhere in the room. Finally the two women put out a few crackers, hoping this would occupy the mouse and keep him quiet for the night.

In the middle of the night she suddenly awoke with an excruciating pain in her left breast. "It was so bad I could hardly breathe," she recounts. But just as suddenly the pain disappeared, and Joan went back to sleep.

The next morning when Joan woke up she hardly remembered the pain until she saw a leftover cracker on the floor. Then the experience came back to her, and with it the memory of pain too severe to be ignored. During the flight home to Minneapolis, the thirty-nine-year-old mother of six thought now and then about the peculiar pain. Barely four months ago she had felt a small lump in that breast; her physician had examined her and said there was nothing to worry about.

Once she was home, Joan wasted no time in talking to her daughter Debbie about the pain. Debbie, a student nurse at the time, was adamant; Joan must be examined again.

On Monday, May 1, Joan saw a different doctor. He, too, was reassuring, and said he felt nothing unusual in the breast. But Joan was not convinced, and she expressed her uneasy concern.

"Well, if it'll make you feel any better, I'll check again," the doctor said.

"When he did," Joan says, "he actually turned red, because this time he did feel the lump. I don't know how long it might have taken to discover my condition had I accepted this doctor's first findings. It's frightening."

Hoping the lump was a cyst, the doctor attempted to aspirate it in his office, but without success. At that point he called a surgeon, and scheduled an examination for Joan that afternoon.

The surgeon's first question was, "Has anybody on your father's side of the family ever had breast cancer?" (The surgeon's emphasis on a history of breast cancer on the paternal side of the family is not shared by the majority of cancer specialists.)

"My grandmother died of breast cancer," Joan replied.

"Then the chances are this is malignant. We'll have to do a biopsy."

Joan's reaction was one of distant unbelief. "I'm the kind of person who can handle a crisis at the time," she explains. "Then afterwards I go to pieces." She left the surgeon's office and drove home to wait for Al.

The timing couldn't have been worse. Al had had a long

day, including a 150-mile round-trip drive to Rochester, Minnesota, for his annual physical at the Mayo Clinic. Moreover, as he drove home he had started to feel sick and weak. When he walked in the house, Joan said, "Honey, I have something to tell you. I'm afraid I have cancer."

"Listen," he said, heading toward the bedroom, "can it wait until tomorrow? I'm sick. I think I'm coming down with the flu."

Joan sat alone after Al went to bed, trying not to worry, trying to understand him, and finally praying. Eventually she was able to sleep.

In the hospital room the following day, Al held Joan's hand as she waited to be wheeled down to the operating room. They prayed together, and, in the Mormon tradition, he gave her a blessing, promising that everything would be all right.

When Joan woke up in the recovery room, the pressure on her chest was so strong it "felt like an elephant sitting there." Gasping for breath, she asked the nearby nurse, "Was it malignant?"

The nurse looked at her with compassion, and said softly, "Yes. They took it all."

"What do you mean, they took it *all?*"

"They did a radical, dear. They took your breast, all the way around to your back."

Shocked, Joan began to cry. She had gone into the operating room believing that the surgeon would do only a biopsy, and that she would be allowed to decide what further surgery should be done if the biopsy showed malignancy.

"That's all right," the nurse comforted her. "Go ahead and cry, honey. Do your crying here, before you get back to your room." Joan did, while the nurse held her hand.

"After I got it out of my system," she says, "I felt better, and then they took me back to my room."

It was a guilt-stricken Al who was ushered in to see her. That morning he had convinced her that the tumor would not

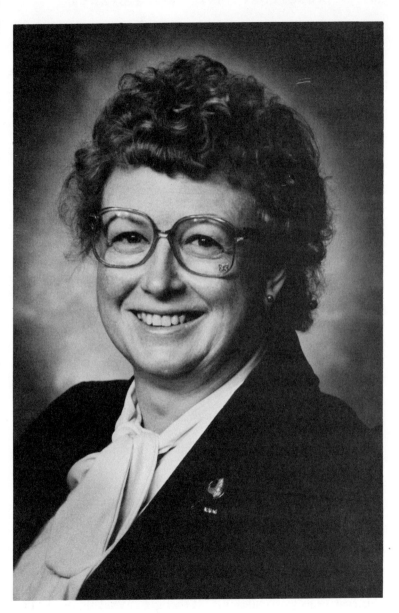

JOAN HEGERMAN

be malignant. Later he had given the permission for the radical. The surgeon, an old-fashioned and strict practitioner, had believed there was no other realistic decision.

Far from blaming Al, however, Joan felt that he should never have been put in that position. "I should have known a great deal more than I did before the biopsy," she says. "I didn't know anything about cancer. In fact, I had a vague impression that once a needle was stuck into the tumor, the cancer could spread all through my body. I mean, I was *ignorant*. I also thought that no matter what the surgeon found, he would just remove the tumor. I never realized a radical mastectomy was a possibility."

It took Joan weeks to convince her husband that she would have made the same decision he did. She was helped by the pathology report on the lymph nodes, which indicated that the cancer had metastasized; that meant a radical probably had been the best procedure. She wasn't helped, however, by the way she received the information from her doctor. Two days after the operation, he came to her door and stood there. "I've got the pathology report," he said gruffly. "It's not good."

Frightened, Joan asked, "What do you mean?"

His expression grim, he said, "I've had pathology reports better than yours on patients who were dead and buried in eighteen months." Then, without another word, he turned and left.

Joan thought that she would explode with fear and anger— terrified by the prognosis and infuriated by the surgeon's insensitivity. But when she calmed down, she began to think about his manner. While most people would view the doctor's behavior as inexcusable, she decided that he was overcome with feelings he could not handle. The more Joan thought about the doctor's prognosis, the more she realized it was self-destructive to worry about it. "I thought, 'What the heck. I'm going to *live* whatever time I have left. There's no sense in worrying myself to death.'"

This did not mean that Joan could forget she'd had cancer—and a negative pathology report. "Sometimes, when the lights were off and I'd said my prayers, I thought about it. But not for long, because I put in a full day, and was always so tired that I fell asleep pretty fast. Being active has been good for me—far better than if I had all kinds of time to sit around and mope."

Even before she was released from the hospital, Joan had resumed her activity. This wasn't difficult, because by its nature her career involves her with thousands of people. Since she and Al started with the Shaklee Corporation in 1962, they have built one of the company's largest distributorships. In the process, Joan has helped develop and motivate thousands of salespeople. Dozens of them came to visit Joan in the hospital, returning some of the caring and sharing they had received from her in the past. In no time her room was effectively converted into an office; when she wasn't visiting with someone, she was on the telephone talking to friends and business associates. And when she wasn't doing that, she was writing letters in answer to those she received from all over the country.

Joan believes that God will sometimes intervene in illness; and she is sure this happened while she was in the hospital. The tubes draining her incisions had plugged up, and she had just been told to expect a minor surgical procedure to insert new tubes. While she lay gloomily wondering how long her healing would take, Al came in with two Elders from the church. They anointed her with oil, put their hands on her head, and blessed her, saying that she would live to see her children raised to maturity. The youngest child was then two, and nothing had bothered Joan more than the thought that she might die before all the children were raised. With the blessing, she experienced both peace and confidence; she felt that cancer was no longer a threat to her—and at that moment the drain tubes began to work again.

In time, Joan achieved an attitude of acceptance about her illness. "I believe there's nothing I can do, other than commit suicide, to hasten my death if it isn't my time to go. If it is, there's nothing I can do to prevent it. I just trust in Heavenly Father, and I live every day He gives me the very best I can."

Joan fully believes that God helps those who help themselves, and by the third day after her surgery, she had decided to help herself. Knowing that she would have to learn to use her left arm all over again, she determined to do as much as she could for herself.

"I wore my hair in a ponytail then, and you can't put up a ponytail with one hand. I made up my mind to manage my hair myself. That was my first goal."

She was sitting in bed with both arms raised, trying to fix her hair, when she looked up to see the surgeon in the door, with a thoroughly shocked expression on his face.

"That's amazing," he said. "I can't believe you're lifting your left arm up and back like that."

The doctor would have been at least as surprised to see Joan in her swimming pool her first day home from the hospital. She was able to swim eight laps that day.

She was accustomed to swimming 132 laps a day, which equaled a mile, in the pool which had been installed for her to use as physical therapy for a chronic hip problem. Born with both hips out of the socket, Joan had received corrective surgery as a toddler. By 1962, however, her hip bones were wearing through into the nerves, and in August of 1963 she had the first of six hip operations. Nothing the doctors could do, though, would correct the noticeable limp resulting from one of the early operations. With her hip problems, her cancer, and other, less major, health problems, Joan has had twenty-one operations in the past nineteen years, some longer and more painful than the mastectomy. Her attitude, again, is accepting—even toward the iatrogenic limp. "I didn't have a limp before I had corrective surgery on my hips," she says, and then adds, tongue-in-cheek, "I guess that's why they call it 'the practice of medicine.' They're still practicing."

A highly confident woman, Joan has not found the psychological aspect of losing a breast too difficult. She deals with the issue with a joke: "I kind of felt I was a lemon to start with. I already had a limp, so I wasn't perfect. What's one more thing?"

Al's reassurance has also helped Joan accept her mastectomy. "He told me over and over that it didn't make any difference to him, that he loved me for *me*, not for what I looked like. It was so important to me to hear that!"

The radical was not without complications. Less than a week after she left the hospital, Joan was readmitted, violently ill. A rapid series of tests showed that her system was rejecting the blood transfusions she had received during the surgery. She recovered from this incident unharmed but frightened. Her fear of another violent reaction led her to reject cobalt and chemotherapy treatment. Somewhat to her surprise, her doctor didn't argue with her.

"That's fine, Joan," he said. "Then we'll skip that."

Joan did not see him again until she went in for her first annual examination. The doctor looked at her strangely, she thought, and during the exam shook his head in disbelief. Finally he stepped back and said, "I just don't believe it."

"Believe what?"

He sighed and admitted to Joan that he had not expected her to live six months, let alone a year. "That's why I didn't object when you refused treatment; I thought you were so far gone it wouldn't have done that much good anyway." He explained that the metastasis to her lymph nodes revealed at the time of her biopsy had led him to deduce there was cancer elsewhere in her body, too. Now, a year later, Joan was active and in good health; and his prognosis was far more positive.

Joan was elated after the visit. She would do what she could to maintain her health. Beyond that, she wanted to forget about cancer. During the seventies she continued to work side by side with her husband building their Shaklee distributorship. In 1980 it included more than twenty-five thousand people, which makes it one of the largest sales forces in the world.

Joan had long been health-conscious, and having had cancer, she made a greater commitment than ever to maintaining good health. In addition to periodic physical examinations, and her daily swim, she's very careful about the food she eats. Her diet consists mainly of fresh fruits and vegetables, chicken and fish (rather than red meat), and whole grains. She uses no discretionary sugar or salt, and takes food supplements religiously: multiple vitamins, vitamin E, sustained-release vitamin C, alfalfa, calcium, and iron. Her three glasses of milk a day are enriched with powdered Instant Protein. Only one thing about Joan's diet is specifically cancer-oriented; she takes laetrile (B-17). She believes all the supplements are good for her, and sees B-17 in the same light. "I don't think laetrile is going to cure cancer all by itself. But I do think it could be beneficial, along with everything else—particularly if you *think* it helps."

Seven years after her mastectomy, Joan realized that wearing a prosthesis was still bothering her. Aware that many women grow comfortable with prosthetic bras, she found hers was always uncomfortable. "It was hot and bothersome in the summer, and in the winter when I put it on—whew, was that thing cold! Add to that the fact that I had to be concerned with it slipping, and I just didn't like it. So I decided to have reconstructive surgery." In 1979 a plastic surgeon performed the operation, which involved the insertion of a plastic bag with saline solution in it. It was not a simple operation, and it included grafting skin from the abdomen onto the breast.

She recovered quickly from this surgery and was soon swimming a mile a day, taking care of her family and the business, and traveling all over America and overseas. In short, she was living the good life.

Then, in June 1981, Joan had a pain in her hip so sharp and sudden that she thought the hip socket might have come loose. She tried to wait it out, since similar pains had come and gone in the past. But this pain was too troubling so she visited her doctor. He assured her there was nothing wrong.

Unsatisfied with this opinion, Joan went to another doctor; he, too, found nothing wrong. Since her experience with her tumor, Joan had learned to be persistent when she felt something wasn't natural. Back she went to the first doctor. This time he sent her to the hospital for tests with a new internist (since her original internist had died). The young doctor was very thorough, and straightforwardly told Joan he believed cancer was the cause of the severe pain. The battery of sophisticated tests he ordered included a CAT scan and a biopsy of a piece of bone from the area where the pain was originating.

The biopsy took place on the eighth day of Joan's hospital confinement. The results showed a nonmalignant tumor in the hip. Joan was inexpressibly relieved when she left the hospital. Two days later she talked to her mother on the telephone, telling her the whole story and reassuring her that everything was fine. When she hung up the receiver, the phone rang. It was the doctor. Unsatisfied with the pathology report, he had sent the bone sample out to two independent laboratories. Both reports had just come back, showing that the tumor was malignant.

Again, Joan had to battle fear and shock. It was worse, perhaps, because she had just been given a clean bill of health. "And then, when my guard was down, they told me I had cancer!"

The medical plan now was for three weeks of daily cobalt treatments, followed by another three weeks of treatment in November. The doctor explained that cobalt would be effective because the malignancy was localized, or confined to one area. The three-minute treatments themselves were painless—but Joan reacted with nausea and extreme diarrhea. "For the first time in my life, I wanted to sleep and sleep and sleep. I was exhausted. I couldn't do much, and I found it almost impossible to keep my spirits up. I missed my work."

This was a new experience for Joan. Even after her radical mastectomy and her extensive hip surgeries she had been able to resume activity almost immediately. Now she could not. It confirmed something she believed, that it was much better for a cancer patient to be involved and active.

"I once read, 'Those who confine themselves to rooms will soon be confined to a room,'" she says. "I learned how true that was. It's just not healthy to sit home with nothing to do but think about how sick you are. You feel much better psychologically when you're concentrating on what's positive about your life.

"Many cancer patients are harmed by gloomy prognoses. I've seen people who were told they had about six months to live, and by golly, in five and a half months, they died! It isn't good to blindly accept the doctor's prognosis; people who do that frame their life around the time they expect to die. After all, doctors aren't God! Just because they predict something doesn't make it so. Yet cancer patients can take a bad prognosis and turn it into a self-fulfilling prophecy."

For Joan, the antidote to anxiety about her cancer-proneness is long-term planning. "Look down the road, and live your life as though you're going to be there!" Even Al sometimes looks doubtful when Joan talks about her long-range goals: seeing her twelve-year-old son graduate from high school; seeing his missionary work for the Mormon Church; attending all the children's weddings. But her philosophy is simple: "If I'm going to be here, I had better make plans for the future. And if I'm not going to be here, it didn't hurt anything to make those plans, did it? Dealing with the future puts you in the stream of life, because this is how you lived before you got cancer. It helps the spirits within, and that helps the healing process."

By nature Joan is an enthusiast who likes to spread the word to others. Her Mormon affiliation enhances this, since the church stresses that each person should be an example for others. For Joan this has meant talking freely to others about her cancer. "It helps people," she says, "because if someday they get cancer, or someone in their family does, they may not be quite so frightened. People are so afraid of cancer today, it's an awful word to most of them. They think having cancer is an automatic death warrant. So I hope that people who see *I* can live with it—and enjoy life, and have a productive and rich life—will understand that they, too, can cope with cancer. The fact that you have cancer doesn't mean you have to roll over and die. I'd like to think I can be an example of that."

Joan incorporates her message into her business talks. She is on the platform primarily to motivate people and tell them how she and Al achieved what they have, and how they can, too. But in each speech she also talks about her bout with cancer. It is part of her overall message: "If I can do it, you can do it, too."

Despite Joan's openness about her cancer, she had to confront the problem of people shying away from her after the recurrence in 1981. The constant requests for speeches dwindled to the point where Joan suspected that many people were avoiding her altogether. Some friends and business associates would call and ask Al how Joan felt, but never ask to talk to her. Others stayed away from her at meetings, as if they felt, "Uh-oh, she got it a second time. Now it's going to be fatal." Joan decided that the only way to get back in the swing of things with the Shaklee organization was to straight-forwardly go out and volunteer to speak. Once she did, people saw that she was the same old Joan, and the speaking engagements once again flowed in.

Joan also felt this fear and avoidance among the women of her church. "They would wave at me, and they'd talk to Al, but it was obvious that they felt uncomfortable around me." Finally she got up the courage to speak out at a women's group. "I'm still me," she said. "I've got cancer, and I'm not afraid to talk about it. I'm not afraid of cancer, or of dying. I'm still going to live my life the same way I lived it before. I'm no different now, except I have something in me that I don't want." The talk was successful in breaking down the barriers that had built up. Once again Joan began to get calls and visits from fellow church members.

Communication with the family during this time went more smoothly. Years before, Joan and Al had established a tradition of family night. Every Monday evening, the whole family joins to discuss household problems, chores, joint deci-sions, and so on. The discussion can range from half an hour to an hour and a half long, and is always followed by what Joan calls "a very sinful dessert," as well as a blessing and a closing prayer. This regular meeting was a natural time to explain Joan's health problems to the children, and to let them air their feelings about her cancer. The openness has helped the family be very supportive of Joan, and she is grateful for the strength that supportiveness gives her. "One thing that's quite important to me," she says, "is that they know better than to give me pity. If all you see is pity, you soon begin to pity yourself."

Joan Hegerman has tackled cancer as she tackles life—with directness and vigor. She makes a point of reading everything she can find about the illness; it gives her a sense of "being armed." She also makes a point of showing those around her that "cancer is not destroying my life, not controlling my whole life. The more I can show that, the more I am an example to other people with serious problems.

"You see," she explains, "that's our reason for being here—to help others, to be an example to them. And knowing that makes it much easier for me to live with cancer."

10

DONNA MYERS

In 1973, when she first suspected she had breast cancer, Donna Myers thought of herself as "the most strappingly healthy woman alive." The attractive forty-seven-year-old wife and mother had every reason to believe her health was excellent. In an area known for its top tennis players, Donna held not one but two top positions that year. She and her partner, Evelyn Robards, were the number one ranked team in the category of Women's 40 Doubles (for women over age forty) in the Northern California Tennis Association (NCTA). And Donna and her husband, Jack, held the NCTA Senior Mixed Doubles title.

Donna's life had reached that enviable point where she was able to involve herself in whatever she wanted to. With the three Myers children enrolled in college, she had cut down her involvement in volunteer organizations and set out to enjoy tennis, bridge, and other activities.

Tennis was Donna's favorite sport. She was competitive and aggressive and a fine athlete. So was her husband. Today a successful executive in the field of auto and truck leasing, Jack Myers was a star fullback for UCLA in the forties. Later he played for the world champion Philadelphia Eagles, and in 1950 was named the team's most valuable player. At age twenty-eight, Jack left pro football to coach at the College of the Pacific, making him the nation's youngest head football coach. Ten years later he retired to begin a career in business.

Jack and Donna began playing tennis to help Donna get back into shape after the birth of their third child. They loved the sport, and were good, and soon were playing "serious" tennis. "I enjoy playing immensely," Donna says, "but I wouldn't play tournaments if Jack didn't. There's no way I'd be away from him all those weekends for tournament tennis. It's only great because we both love it. Jack is an angel—I adore him—and if he were into golf, then I'd play golf instead of tennis."

It was Jack who first felt a tiny lump on Donna's left breast in June of 1973. Donna was able to feel the lump, too, but was not frightened by it. "How could I possibly have cancer?" she thought. "I feel so good!" She also thought there was no history of cancer in her family. Still, it was just good sense to make an appointment with the internist.

His evaluation was reassuring. The lump was very small, and was located in the inner quadrant of the breast, both good signs. The lump could be any of at least ten things, nine of which were benign. "It doesn't fit any of the criteria for cancer," the doctor told her. "Let's watch it for six months."

Donna felt wonderful, and went on with her life as before, with no anxiety about the small, seemingly harmless lump.

In December, as scheduled, she returned to the doctor for a follow-up. He had made careful notes of the exact size of the lump on the first visit. Now he said, "Donna, I don't think it's anything, but I do see some change. It's a very slight change, but I'd recommend you see a surgeon."

Donna made an appointment with a surgeon who is a close friend of the family. After a thorough examination, he said that he, too, thought it was not malignant—but he wanted Donna to have a biopsy taken.

Donna was unworried, and her main concern was that the family enjoy Christmas without the children being unduly worried. "I asked if we couldn't wait another two weeks, until the children left after Christmas, and everyone thought that would be okay." The day the children left to return to their schools, Donna was admitted to El Camino Hospital.

Calm and confident as she was, even Donna was momentarily shaken when the hospital asked her to sign papers giving the surgeon permission to remove her breast if the biopsy showed malignancy. She signed the release, and shrugged off her brief fear. "I'm not a hysterical person," she explains. "And I fully believed it was benign." In this frame of mind, she went under the anesthetic.

She awoke in her hospital room to find Jack holding her hand. "Honey, I have something to tell you," he said gently.

Donna remembered something she overheard—or thought she overheard—while unconscious in the operating room. "You don't have to tell me," she said. "I don't have my breast. I know it."

"That's right," Jack said. "You don't."

The tumor had been malignant; the surgeon had performed a mastectomy.

The doctors told Donna and Jack that the cancer had been entirely removed and that she had nothing more to worry about. "The only people I'd ever known who had mastectomies had died: Jack's older cousin and a neighbor. So I had the impression that people just didn't live long after breast cancer. I was glad to be told otherwise."

Armed with this good news, Donna was prepared to tell the children about the surgery. "I told them I was okay," she says, "and they believed me because they know I try always to be honest and open. So I was minus a breast, but there was no cancer in the lymph nodes and everything would be fine. I

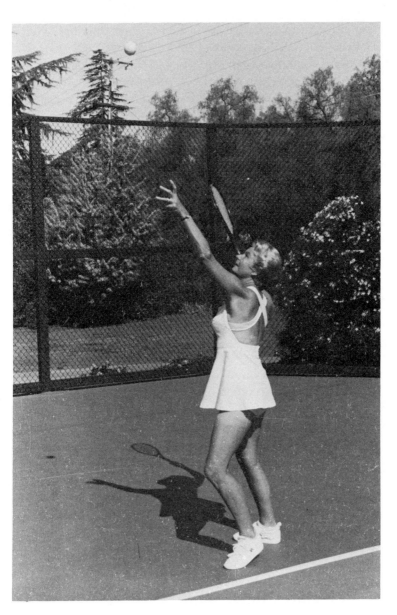

DONNA MYERS

wanted them to hear that from me, so they wouldn't be up-set." From her room, Donna and Jack called Clyde, their older son, at his college in Oregon, and then Marilee, who was living in the area. Both children asked numerous questions, and the Myerses talked to them until they were reassured. Their second son, Jack, found out when he came home unex-pectedly while Donna was still in the hospital. Donna's good spirits reassured him, too. Throughout, Donna's only real anxiety had been for the children. Now that they were com-fortable with the news, she really did feel great. Four days after her surgery she was discharged from the hospital.

"I drove my car that same day," she admits. "I felt so well that it didn't occur to me not to."

As far as Donna was concerned, the only real problem with the mastectomy was that she could not play tennis at the moment. The day she left the hospital, she asked the doctor, "Hey, when can I play tennis?"

With a grin he replied, "Knowing you, you'll be out there next week."

Donna knew that he was kidding, but, she says, "After all, the mastectomy was on my left side, and I am right-handed." The next week she met three women friends at her club, as usual, for tennis, lunch, and an afternoon of bridge. Still stitched and bandaged, Donna had no idea if she really could play. When she stepped onto the court, she was not in pain, but she thought pain might build up. "But it felt great!" she says, "just great! They kept asking if I was okay, and finally I said, 'Hey, forget it, let's play!' And we played three sets that day."

Before he saw Donna again, her surgeon learned through mutual friends that she had been out playing tennis seven days after her surgery. "My God," he said to her, "who told you that you could do that?"

"Well, you did," Donna laughed.

"I didn't *mean* it."

"I thought you did," Donna kidded, "but don't worry, I'm fine."

Donna was fine, and she was back into her old routine. In her mind, it had been a minor skirmish with cancer. There was one major effect: life was enhanced by her realization of how lucky she had been. "They examined all the lymph nodes, and none of them had a trace of cancer. What's more, if I'd had that biopsy six months sooner, I might have had a radical mastectomy instead of a modified. It was just during that time that the doctors in my area changed to the less drastic procedure. And a radical would have really affected my mobility. The other piece of good fortune was the kind of breast cancer I had. Out of about six types, I had infiltrating ductile carcinoma, which seldom occurs in the other breast. That meant I didn't have to worry about follow-up treatment, but could be checked periodically for possible recurrence."

A happy woman, Donna proceeded to purchase a prosthesis and plunge back into her life. She was pleased to find that many rumors about mastectomies were untrue; she could wear all the clothes she usually wore. "In fact, they make such great prostheses now that if I kept my big mouth shut, nobody would even know I'd had a mastectomy. I'm not the kind to keep a secret, though, and I never cared who knew."

Before the operation, Donna gave little thought to the possibility that she might lose a breast and the effect it might have on her husband. It did cross her mind that a mastectomy could have a profound negative effect on Jack, but that was only a fleeting thought. "After all, I knew my husband and felt completely secure about our relationship. I was right, of course; nothing changed between us after the operation. Jack convinced me, mostly by the way he treated me, that I was the same total person as before and that he still loved me."

Soon Donna's tennis was as good as ever. In 1975 she and Evelyn were ranked as the number one team in the country in Women's Senior Doubles. It was the eighth consecutive year they had ranked in the top seven in this category, an achievement enhanced by the fact that Donna, at age forty-nine, was competing against women in their early forties. The partners had also been number one in the NCTA for six of those eight years.

Donna had put all thoughts of cancer behind her when, in June 1975, Jack thought that he felt a very small lump in her breast. Donna went to the internist immediately.

Even with the use of a mammogram, the doctor was hardly able to detect the minute lump. With that, and the fact that Donna's cancer was not a type that recurs in the other breast, he felt there was nothing to worry about. "Let's check again in three months," he said.

Relieved, Donna agreed, and went out to play the tournament season. In September, a checkup showed the tiny lump hadn't changed. Three months later, it still seemed unchanged. However, Donna's history prompted the doctor to say, "Look, this is ridiculous. This lump is close to the surface, it's tiny, there's no sense in your making all these visits. Let's get this out under local anesthetic, as an outpatient, and then we'll know, and that'll be the end of it."

"Great," Donna concurred.

The same surgeon did the simple lumpectomy, while Donna chatted away about tennis. "Doesn't look like anything to worry about," he told her. "I'll call you tonight with the results of the biopsy."

When he called that evening, Donna instantly knew that something was terribly wrong; his voice cracked as he told her, "Donna, it's another primary tumor. It has nothing to do with your first one, so it's not a recurrence—that's good news. The bad news is that you've got another kind of cancer. Donna . . . we're going to have to do another mastectomy."

Not able to deal with the reality of his words, Donna cried out, "I'm just leaving for a national tournament. The draw has been made, and we're seeded. I have to go."

"You cannot go."

"I *have* to."

"I'm sorry, Donna, but this time you can't. We're talking about saving your life here. You've got to get in the hospital this Monday for the mastectomy."

Shocked and depressed, Donna had a hard time accepting this sudden intrusion into her life. Losing a second breast was much more traumatic than losing the first. "Sure, I already wore a prosthesis. But I felt that as long as one of my breasts was my own, I wasn't really cheating. *One* was mine. But now . . . well, I got the blues that night."

By Monday, though, Donna was joking and making light of the problem with two friends who came with her to the hospital. The three women had fallen into giggling over the possibilities of a full prosthesis. "I can be any size now," Donna was saying. "Can you picture me as Dolly Parton?"

Just then an aide entered the room with a wheelchair, and told Donna he was to take her for more X rays. Instantly she was wary; upon entering the hospital she had taken the necessary blood tests and X rays, and she remembered that the X rays had been developed and checked before she was allowed to leave. "Something must be wrong," she thought.

The new test, a topography, did nothing to reassure her. As she held still for the repeated X rays of the layers of her body, which homed in on specific areas of her chest, Donna studied the faces of the X-ray technicians. Their expressions seemed very somber to her.

After the tests, upset and frightened, Donna was wheeled back to her room. Jack and the surgeon were there. By their expressions she was positive that something was really wrong.

"What is it?" she asked.

The doctor explained that although they never expected a recurrence of her initial cancer, they knew that it was within the realm of possibility. It could progress from the breast to the bones and then the lungs, and it could do this about two years after the mastectomy. It seemed likely now that that was what had happened. The X rays showed a spot on Donna's lung and everything indicated the first cancer had recurred.

That night Donna fell asleep trying not to think about the new threat. Instead of having a mastectomy in the morning, she was scheduled for new tests, including full body bone scans. The mastectomy would be done only if the scans showed that the cancer had not metastasized to her bones.

For Donna, the day of being rolled around on a gurney for testing was strange and unreal. Tanned and fit, she looked perfectly healthy, and felt wonderful. "It's just incredible that I could be sick," she thought.

When the radiologist finally came up with the results, he said to Donna, "I've got good news."

"You mean I get to have a mastectomy?"

Donna laughs as she recalls the scene. "I was so happy to think I would just have a mastectomy—because it meant there was no cancer in my bones. The staff at the hospital said Christmas came a little early for me that year!"

Before she had assimilated the good news, Donna was wheeled into the operating room and placed under anesthesia. When she woke up, she had had her second mastectomy. It seemed a minor concern, compared to the mysterious spot on her lung. In the next twenty-four hours she lost track of the number of people who came to her room to ask questions that might help identify the spot on her lung. Valley fever was suspected. Donna had played in tournaments in the San Joaquin valley, where there had been an outbreak. But, she protested, people died of valley fever, and she had never even felt sick. The physician told her some people who contracted the disease never even knew it. But a serum injection came up negative, indicating that Donna had never had valley fever. After that, she was tested for every possible cause of the spot; each test came up negative.

Her case was finally brought up before a tumor board of

nine physicians, who reviewed her entire history. Each member then wrote his or her own recommendation. The recommendation of the board was unanimous: since nobody could determine the cause of the spot, Donna should have thoracic surgery to have it removed.

The thoracic surgeon showed Donna and Jack the X ray and pointed out the spot, just under the incision where Donna's right breast had been removed. Its position was good, he said; because it was on the outside edge of the lung, it would not be necessary to remove the entire upper lobe. He added, "Everybody agrees that there's a 99 percent probability this is malignant. If you don't have it removed, we're going to have to run all those tests every couple of months to keep tabs on it. I strongly recommend you have the surgery."

"I suppose I don't have any choice," Donna said with a sigh. "But I want to know all the ramifications of the operation."

The surgeon took Donna and Jack into his private office, closed the door, and read to them two pages of information detailing the possible results of thoracic surgery. "It got kind of hairy," Donna says. "It told how your lung might collapse, everything."

But she and Jack agreed that so many doctors must be right, and the operation was scheduled.

This time the situation was considered too serious to let Donna wait until after the holidays. Just before Christmas she was once again wheeled into the operating room. The thoracic surgery was much more extensive than the mastectomies had been; it entailed removing part of one rib, as well as a wedge-shaped section of lung which included the spot. The aftermath of the operation was also more painful for Donna, who spent the first twenty-four hours of her recovery in an intensive care unit. But the news was good. The spot was not malignant. What it was, the doctors did not immediately know; it would take the lab three days to diagnose it.

The third day after the operation, Donna was getting ready

to leave the hospital when the doctor came in with the news. The lab tests showed that the spot on her lungs had been caused by nothing other than valley fever.

"I almost fell off the bed!" Donna says. "That meant I didn't have to have that operation at all.

"But I learned something from that. I had been tested for valley fever, and it tested negative. I think people assume that tests are 100 percent accurate, but few of them are. That test showed negative, when I'd actually had the disease. To give you another example, mammograms are a wonderful diagnostic tool, but they're only about 80 percent accurate. The important thing about that is, if a woman's mammogram is negative, that doesn't mean she's home free. If she has a lump, she should still watch it carefully, and have it checked regularly."

Donna is no complainer, but even she says "the thoracic surgery was horrendous. The mastectomies were nothing compared to that." Before the operation she had been told she could not play tennis for at least three months, and possibly six months. Two weeks after surgery, however, when she returned to the doctor for a checkup, he discovered her rib had already begun to regrow.

"You can start hitting tennis balls again," he told her.

"Hey, I don't *have* to play tennis," Donna said, acutely aware of the fact that she had two incisions healing, one of which went entirely around her right side.

"You're healing so fast I'm afraid you'll get adhesions. Go out and hit tennis balls."

"I couldn't believe it!" Donna says enthusiastically, "and neither could Jack. When I came home and told him, I practically had to hit him with a brick to make him believe it."

When hitting tennis balls, she had to be careful not to raise her arm. In minutes, Donna learned that it didn't hurt. So she gathered up some friends, hit everything underhand, served underhand—and played tennis. Ten weeks later the doctor told her she could raise her arm when she played. A few days after that, she and Evelyn won a Women's Senior Doubles tournament!

While cancer did not slow Donna Myers down, it did change her life—in some very positive ways. Soon after her lung surgery, she sat down to do some serious self-analysis. "I decided I was obviously doing something wrong with my life. So far I'd been lucky, but another bout with cancer could be disastrous. So I decided to learn about what I should be doing."

Donna read everything she could about breast cancer and went to a meeting of the local cancer society. At that meeting, a small event moved her life in a new direction. A woman there asked if Donna would model in a fashion show to be held by Reach to Recovery, an organization whose volunteer members work with breast cancer patients. Donna agreed. The show introduced her to "a wonderful group of girls, and a great program. I decided to put aside some of the fun things I was doing, and use that time to help other women overcome the trauma of a mastectomy."

As a Reach to Recovery volunteer, Donna was trained in every aspect of reaching out to help a new mastectomy patient. This meant being knowledgeable, since "most women are on square one in terms of what they know about a mastectomy, even with all the publicity on breast cancer today. People think it's something that can never happen to them." Donna talks to a patient by phone before visiting, and always enters a room with the Reach to Recovery spirit: "Looking good and feeling good. That's so important. Just the fact that we come in looking healthy and happy, and we have complete mobility—that does wonders for a patient's morale." Donna talks to the women she helps about clothing and prostheses, and sometimes shares her own experiences with her mastectomies when she feels that will be of some value. She is not a shy person, and has modeled and appeared on television numerous times to show women that a woman can look good after two mastectomies.

"In fact," she says, her face lighting up, "I look better. I do! When I went to get my second prosthesis, I took a good friend who is an excellent judge of fit and proportion. Well, we spent over two hours in that dressing room, and we laughed ourselves sick! I realized that now I could be any size, so I tried on all kinds of things.

"I finally decided that even my first prosthesis was too heavy—it was a 34D, to match my right breast—so I went a size smaller. And I've been so happy with it. I can wear strapless dresses, halters, all kinds of things I never could wear before, when I was larger."

When she models, Donna is usually wearing clothes made by Keddie Kreations, a manufacturer which has designed special outfits for her to model at American Cancer Society shows. "These low-cut dresses are more revealing and outlandish than I used to wear before my mastectomies," Donna says with a bright laugh. "We've dreamed up all kinds of backless, strapless things just to show what can be done. You can't believe how that delights women!"

Donna looks so natural in her prosthesis that she is often asked whether she has had reconstruction. She has not. "In my case, the surgery would have been so extensive that I was afraid I'd lose some mobility and my tennis would be affected. Jack doesn't care, so it isn't important to me." In a recent speech, she shared her philosophy on this subject. "I have not been reconstructed and have no plans to be. I feel just as normal today as I did when I had breasts. I can do everything I did before, and equally as well. I am the same person, with the same self-esteem. Femininity is a state of mind. Being loving, giving, involved, perceptive, and accepting are human qualities that make me feel feminine."

For many women, Donna adds, reconstruction is wonderful. "I know women who are very happy with it. It's an individual decision, and a woman should just be sure she understands her condition and the options." At monthly Reach to Recovery meetings, the options in prostheses are displayed and explained to anyone who is interested. "We always have outstanding speakers—surgeons, oncologists, dietitians, people in all kinds of related fields. I know for me these talks are so helpful; I always learn something more about breast cancer."

As the name implies, Reach to Recovery shows mastectomy patients how to use stretching exercises to regain their strength and mobility. Donna explains, "It would be ridiculous for me to urge a woman to get out and play tennis as I did. Tennis just happens to be my thing. But my message to them is that they *can* get back into their lives, that someday they, too, can do whatever they used to do."

Donna's message is conveyed as much by her active life as by her words. One patient, who had been an excellent horsewoman and competed in shows, told Donna recently: "I've been sitting around feeling sorry for myself—but I can't help seeing what you've done with your tennis. I said to myself, 'If Donna could do it, I know darn well I can do it.' I'm going to start riding again."

Donna's achievements since her mastectomies have been astounding. In 1978, when she was fifty-two years old, she and Evelyn were ranked number one in both Women's 40 and Women's 50 categories by the NCTA—the first time any team had won both honors simultaneously. They repeated that feat in 1981, when she was fifty-five. Donna and Jack ranked number one in the NCTA's Senior Mixed Doubles (for women over forty and men over forty-five) that year, the second time they had earned that spot (the other time was in 1973). Ever since, Donna has continued to earn high rankings. In the U.S. Tennis Association, she was number three in Women's 50 Doubles in 1980; in 1982 she was runner-up for the National Women's 50 Doubles indoor title.

The Myers trophy room gives physical proof of how rewarding tennis has been to Donna. Still, Donna says she is finding her work for Reach to Recovery more fulfilling than anything she's ever done before.

"All my life I've been an active person, very people-oriented. I'd done a lot of public speaking and community work, and everything I did gave me a little skill and expertise in something new. But in Reach to Recovery I'm able to take all those skills and use them to help other people. I've progressed to being an area consultant, so I help solve problems and upgrade the program in twelve northern California counties. It may sound funny, but I understand what people mean when they say they found their calling in life. I get an inner satisfaction from what I do now that I've never found anywhere else.

"I'm still surprised that I've had cancer. I guess the toughest thing was having to face the fact that it did happen to me. It really has made me aware of the importance of each day, and I think that is good. I know I get more value out of my days now."

Donna doesn't minimize the serious trauma of a mastectomy. "I'm not saying I didn't like my breasts. I did," she emphasizes. "And I'd like to have them back. However, I can't. But the truth is that losing a finger would have handicapped me more as a tennis player than losing a breast; it would have been disabling. And losing a breast is not disabling—unless you let it defeat you mentally."

Today, at age fifty-six, Donna looks and feels at least ten years younger. She still excels at tennis, routinely besting opponents several years younger than herself. From the other side of the net, Donna Myers looks like a healthy, strong, and worthy adversary, and she is. She refuses to be defeated, on the court—or off.

11

BRENDA MUSSER

In March 1975 Brenda was twenty-eight, single, and doing things with her life. She was successfully operating a beauty salon with eight employees and had recently signed a five-year lease with a large downtown hotel in Columbus, Ohio. Now she was preparing to open a boutique in the same hotel. Financing both businesses had put her in debt, but she was confident she would make it.

Her life was just what she wanted it to be—except, lately, she was tired too much of the time. At first she blamed it on the long hours she worked and the pressure and anxiety of setting up a new business. Soon the fatigue became a serious problem. She could barely make it through the day, and woke up in the morning as tired as if she hadn't slept. Brenda decided to see her doctor.

The examination revealed a swollen lymph gland in Brenda's neck. While the doctor speculated that her fatigue was probably caused by anemia, he also suggested she enter the hospital for "some routine tests." Brenda was reluctant, since the boutique was due to open in less than two weeks. Still, she agreed, thinking that whatever the tests showed, the bedrest would be good for her.

There was no doubt in Brenda's mind that she was a healthy person. She had worked too hard, she thought, and was now paying for it. So she was stunned when the doctor told her that the tests showed that she had Hodgkin's disease, a form of cancer affecting the lymphatic system.

Her shock turned to terror. She became so hysterical that the nurses gave her a shot to calm her down. "It took two hours before I got back my composure," she says. "I was still scared, but the panic was gone.

"I had to get in touch with my family, and that worried me. My mother had heart problems and high blood pressure, and I couldn't deal with the idea that the news might cause something bad to happen to her. When I was calm enough, I called my older sister, who lives in Kentucky near my parents. She and her husband went to break the news to my mother. I knew my mother would be calling me, and I wanted to find some way to distract her. I decided to ask her to prepare a meal for me and I designed a menu so complicated that I knew it would take all her energy just to buy the food and prepare everything. It really worked, but like most distractions it was only temporary."

In the months to come Brenda found that her mother had more difficulty adjusting than she did. "Whenever she would visit me," Brenda explains, "she'd try so hard not to cry, but she always would. It helped me, as it turned out, because I knew the only way I could make her feel better was to *get* better. It firmed up my resolve to beat this thing."

Seven days after she received the diagnosis of cancer, Brenda underwent a splenectomy (the removal of her spleen). She agreed to have the surgeon tie her Fallopian tubes during the operation because the proposed course of treatment included cobalt therapy, which would affect her ovaries and greatly reduce her chances of bearing healthy children.

During the next eighteen weeks Brenda had sixty cobalt treatments. Each one took only a few minutes. "You just lie

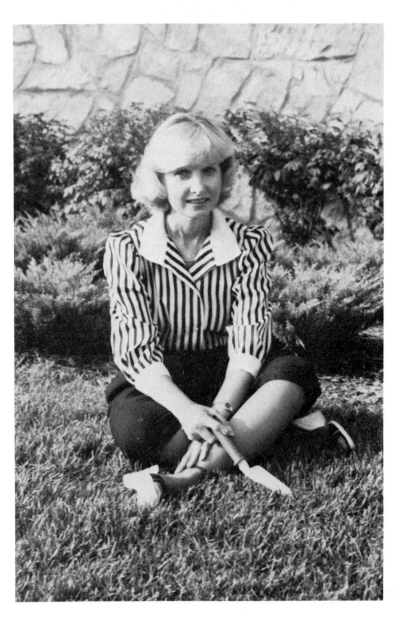

BRENDA MUSSER

on a table and they turn on the machine and you sing a song," Brenda says lightly. "Then you get up and go home." Spared the nausea and diarrhea that sometimes accompany cobalt treatments, Brenda did suffer burns on her chest which left permanent scars. She shrugs. "I can't wear low-cut dresses or swim suits anymore. I wish I could . . . but it's no big deal."

Brenda knew that cobalt therapy can also cause hair loss. For any woman this can be devastating.

"Sometimes I worried about it all night," she says. "A woman's hair *is* her crowning glory, and especially in my business. I trembled at the thought of myself in the salon, bald, around all those people who are in there to make their hair and skin beautiful. It seems strange now, but I was much more upset over the possibility of losing my hair than I was over the certainty that I would never be able to bear a child. I can't explain it; maybe I was so worried about staying alive that I couldn't think ahead to a time when I might marry and want children. Maybe, somehow, I connected losing my hair with losing my life—and that terrified me then."

Brenda did lose hair high on the back of her head; so she designed a hair style to cover the baldness. It was so effective that more than one customer thought it was a new French hair style.

She told anyone who asked about it, "It came all the way from my hospital. They were having a special."

While the salon thrived, the boutique stayed open only a year. Brenda simply wasn't up to running two businesses. She had only a fraction of her normal stamina, and not nearly enough strength to make the frequent buying trips to New York needed to build the boutique.

Her doctors suggested she get out of the beauty salon business. Anyone who has cancer, they said, should stay away from sprays and chemicals. Brenda understood that their advice was prudent, but after much thought she decided not to get out of the business. First of all, she was in debt for the business. She would have faced financial ruin if she had closed it. Secondly, the beauty business was not only her specialty, and her living, it was also something she loved, something she got great rewards from. At her salon she was surrounded by hairdressers and clients who knew of her illness and supported her. And the bright, single woman needed all the support she could get.

Because Brenda believed that word of her illness would spread throughout her clientele no matter what she did, she was completely open about it.

"Most people were wonderful," she says, "and no matter how I felt, I acted cheerful. Being positive was the way to get well again. And the way to keep my customers."

Although Brenda freely talked about her illness, she was occasionally irritated by people who assumed very somber, worried expressions around her. "They'd come up to me as if I were on my deathbed," she says, "with their heads down. Then they'd look up through their eyebrows and say in such a pitying way, 'Oh Brenda, how *are* you?' To tell you the truth, I wanted to hit them! But what I would do was ask them, 'How do I look?'

"Well! What can they say—'You look terrible'? Never! So they'd tell me I looked great, and I'd say, 'Good!' And that would be that. Pretty soon they'd forget I had a problem.

"It's easy to crawl in a hole and pity yourself. I know some people just give up when they're seriously ill. I really don't understand that attitude. They seem to give in to the idea that they're going to die. I believe in making my peace with death and then getting up and showing the world that I'm alive. My work helped me a great deal. I faced people every day. My livelihood depended on being cheerful. That gave me a real incentive!"

Although Brenda knew how important a positive attitude was to recovery, she often had to battle depression. "Some mornings I woke up feeling great and forgot for a few moments that I had Hodgkin's disease. Then it would come crashing in on me. Rejecting the disease was something I had to fight. I *had* to accept it; it happened to me. God wasn't punishing me for something I did. It just happened, that's all. And I reminded myself I wasn't going to be the last person who had Hodgkin's. I'd say to myself, 'You've got it, Brenda, but you better get on with your life.'"

Her doctor, Thomas Nims, was always straightforward and honest about the illness, the treatment, and the rate of recovery. "I believe that if I didn't trust him," she says, "my body would not have responded so well to those treatments. Tom always dealt with me realistically, and I could handle that. I'm grateful that he didn't treat me like a weak sister and try to pacify me with things that weren't true. His approach made it possible for me to participate in my healing. And a patient's participation is essential."

She is certain that she wouldn't have overcome her cancer without skilled medical care. "But I had a lot to do with my recovery," she adds. "It's like a marriage; one partner can't do it all. If the patient and the doctors don't work together, the odds aren't nearly as good."

Her sickness has made Brenda more philosophical. She began studying the Bible closely for the first time in her life. After reading a text or parable, she would close her eyes and meditate on the meaning of it, using the scripture to "pull everything together." She used this time to review her day and think about how she might act differently the next day. "It worked well for me," she says. "I'd come up with some very nice thoughts, and often felt peaceful and calm afterward. It was important that I relax—listening to soft music, practicing yoga exercises and meditating really helped me."

Brenda kept a written record of her goals, both short- and long-term, and religiously monitored her progress. She had always had "a burning desire to *be* somebody" and was determined not to let her illness stop her. "Those ambitions were good for me," she says. "There were times when that's what kept me going. I still put everything down on paper, for what I want out of life to what I want to accomplish today. I have weekly, monthly, and annual lists, and as I do things I check them off. On paper I work through my feelings and my problems."

Although she has no desire to be a writer, Brenda has written hundreds of pages during her convalescence. The resultant manuscript she calls "a six-year diary of life with cancer."

"When I read over what I have written, I know that things were never as bad as I thought," she says. "Sometimes things I thought were awful were actually amusing. Writing it all down worked for me. It was like being angry with someone and writing an angry letter in which you really ream them out. You read the letter and then tear it up—you've got it all out of your system. That's what my writing down unhappy thoughts did for me."

During those times when she felt really depressed, she would find a place to be alone and let herself cry. "I mean a really good cry that comes from down in my soul," she says earnestly. "I'd just let the tears come and stream down my face. And no matter how mean and grumpy I might have been, I always felt good after I cried. I'd get up and fix my face, and my whole attitude would be changed."

Brenda's new life included regular church attendance. And she joined the American Medical Federation, which is considered extremist by some because of its emphasis on nutrition. "We believe in medical treatment; but we also believe that people who practice positive thinking and supplement their diets with vitamins don't need as much medical treatment as they otherwise would."

Brenda doesn't rely on food supplements for nourishment. She is careful to follow a healthy, well-balanced diet, and uses little or no sugar, salt, or refined white flour. Her diet is made up of fruits, vegetables, fish, and chicken, with only moderate amounts of red meat. "Eating well," she says, "takes time and organization." At first she had to spend a lot of each weekend shopping, preparing meals, and counting out each day's vitamins for the week ahead, but now these chores take less time. Her daily routine includes plenty of exercise—calisthenics, long walks, and aerobic dancing—but Brenda has also learned to indulge her body's need for rest.

Brenda did not feel handicapped in her battle with cancer because she was single and lived alone. "Maybe it was to my advantage. I could completely close myself away from the world and collect my thoughts, without any interruptions. I didn't have to worry about anybody else. I could concentrate on defeating my cancer.

"There were times, of course, when being alone hurt," Brenda says. "Sometimes, in the middle of the night, I wasn't quite sure I would live until morning. I was afraid to go to sleep—afraid that I might not wake up. So I'd turn on the TV and sit up and watch it all night. It might have been easier if I had somebody at times like that. But I didn't."

Brenda has somebody now. Russell Musser. The two met and married in 1979. Brenda found when she married Russ that her inability to bear children mattered far more now than it had when she had agreed to have her tubes tied. "Russ reminded me once that under certain circumstances the type of operation I had could be reversed. But I remembered what the doctors told me about my chances of ever bearing a healthy child. They scared me so much, I didn't give the operation much thought. I regret not being able to bear children, but I know I made the right choice."

Recovery from cancer is seldom a straight, upward path with no temporary defeats. Many patients experience remission, only to be disappointed by a later setback. While Brenda had no recurrence of Hodgkin's disease, in 1977 she did experience a side effect of cobalt therapy so serious it threatened her life. Due to a complex and unique mechanical failure, Brenda was subjected to excessive radiation, which caused internal scar tissue to form. Two years after her therapy, the tissue moved and caused constrictive pericarditis, so that her pericardium (the sac around the heart) filled with fluid. The fluid retention spread to the rest of her body, until at its worst the diameter of her left upper arm measured six and a half inches larger than that of her right arm, and her feet were so swollen she could hardly walk. This edema came on with dizzying rapidity. Before Brenda knew what was happening, she was literally drowning in her own fluids.

Admitted to a Columbus hospital, Brenda was given a battery of tests over a period of eighteen days. "When the results came in, the doctors insisted I was experiencing a recurrence of cancer and must have surgery. They told me that in cases like mine, cancer could cause my arms and legs to swell up like that, but that didn't make any sense to me. I refused to accept the diagnosis. I knew in my heart I didn't have cancer."

Looking for support Brenda called her original doctor, Tom Nims, who had taken a leave of absence to work at Sloan-Kettering in New York City. After discussing the situation with him, she decided not to have the operation.

Hanging up the phone, Brenda told the startled nurse that she was checking out.

While Brenda packed, the nurse left the room, then returned to say, "I called the staff doctor to tell him what you're doing. He says to tell you that if you sign out, you'll have to find a new physician."

Even though she acted assertively, Brenda's confidence was shaky as she walked out of the hospital. "I kept wondering, 'Is it possible that all these doctors are wrong?' I kept remembering my first reaction when I was told I had cancer; I didn't want to accept it then, either."

In searching for a doctor she would have full confidence in,

Brenda remembered the experience of a friend who had had lung cancer and had been given three months to live. He had gone to an M.D. in Michigan who used the thermoscan to confirm the presence or absence of cancer. The thermoscan uses body heat to show what's going on in the patient's body; it is considered unorthodox by many physicians.

"It worked," Brenda says. "In five hours that doctor told me what those other doctors hadn't figured out in eighteen days. There was no cancer at all. What I had was constrictive pericarditis."

Back home in Columbus, Brenda went to a holistic practitioner, who prescribed natural foods, vitamins, and exercise in addition to conventional medical treatments. "I thought that he was wonderful," she says. "He was almost eighty years old, and he jogged every day, and he could run circles around people half his age. His concepts were great. The only trouble was, I kept right on swelling."

Finally Brenda was so ill she went home to Pikeville, Kentucky, where her mother could care for her. The fluid was so bad now that it became more and more difficult for her to breathe.

By Thanksgiving Day Brenda was so ill that her mother insisted they go to the local hospital. As she walked Brenda to the car Brenda insisted, "I will *not* go another round with these doctors. I'd rather die."

But the trip to the small emergency room was the best medical decision yet. There Brenda met Dr. Bill Hambley, mayor of Pikeville, former law student, and a physician experienced in everything from delivering babies to performing brain surgery. Bill Hambley was very troubled when the dying young woman walked in. Vaguely Brenda heard him say to her mother, "If she makes it through the night, we stand a chance." To Brenda, in a fog of pain, the words were not upsetting. "It was like watching a movie and hearing that said about someone else. I wasn't emotionally involved."

Dr. Hambley prescribed albumin treatments for his new patient, giving the first ones in veins in the groin, since her arms were so swollen he could not locate the veins. Brenda did survive the night, and the next day felt significantly better. The albumin treatments were providing proteins her liver was now unable to produce, due to the effects of cobalt therapy.

By her fourth day she was feeling relatively spunky. And in the next ten days, she lost fifteen pounds of excess water. Since then, Brenda has had no recurrence of either cancer or pericarditis. Her original surgeon, Tom Nims, has confirmed that she never did have a recurrence of cancer after her Hodgkin's disease in 1975. The only therapy she receives today is periodic albumin treatments.

While statistics indicate that the average individual's life expectancy is shortened by a bout with cancer, Brenda believes her life span will be normal. "Since I've had cancer," she says, "I'm aware of my body and I take care of it. If I feel pain, I think, 'I better see a doctor.' I get enough rest, I eat well, I exercise. Once you've been really sick, these things become part of your life. They are part of my life now—and they will stay with me a long time because I intend to live a long time."

12

RICHARD BLOCH

In November 1977 Dick and Annette Bloch were happily ensconced in a rented villa in Acapulco. Between trips such as this one and visits to their home in Fort Lauderdale, the couple managed to avoid the worst of the cold Kansas City winters. The "R" in H & R Block, Dick had founded the tax preparation chain in 1955 with his brother Henry, and built the company until, with more than nine thousand offices, it was the largest of its kind in the world. Now semiretired, the chairman of the board was enjoying the good life.

The Blochs' first week in Acapulco was only slightly marred by Dick's stiff neck. It was more of a nuisance than anything, and he attributed it to either his daily tennis or the villa's air conditioning. By the time the Blochs returned to Kansas City, the discomfort had migrated to Dick's shoulder. He called a doctor, who X-rayed the shoulder and assured Dick it was a minor muscular problem.

"That's a relief," Dick said. "It reminded me of a pain in the shoulder my uncle complained about, before he died of cancer."

This information renewed the doctor's concern about the

situation. He took three more X-rays of the shoulder before he was satisfied. "It's definitely not cancer. The soreness should be gone within a month." Dick was glad to take such a positive diagnosis to Annette, whom he now told for the first time of the persistent pain.

The couple vacationed in Florida during the month of January, but Dick's shoulder, instead of healing, was getting worse, and the pain was now extending down his right arm. As soon as he was back in Kansas City, Dick went to an orthopedic surgeon, who told him the previous doctor had X-rayed the wrong part of the body. After X-raying Dick's neck, the orthopedic surgeon concluded that arthritis in the neck was rubbing a nerve.

After the Blochs returned to their house in Florida, however, the pain increased again. It was accompanied by a frightening numbness that grew until Dick could no longer grip anything firmly with his right hand. In late March, back home in Kansas City again, he called a second orthopedic surgeon, who listened to Dick's description of his symptoms and told him to call a neurosurgeon. The neurosurgeon's reaction to the story was quick and to the point; he told Dick to meet him within an hour at the emergency room of the hospital he worked through.

Among the first questions the neurosurgeon asked Dick was if he smoked. "No," Dick replied. "And I don't like that question." The doctor shrugged.

At 7:30 the next morning, the hospital laboratory began running tests. A chest X ray revealed a large mass on the upper segment of Dick's right lung. A bone scan confirmed that the mass was a tumor. The neurosurgeon scheduled Dick for a biopsy the next morning.

To Annette and the Blochs' three daughters, the biopsy seemed to take forever. As they sat in the waiting room, they tried to deal with the possibility that the tumor might be malignant. From the moment Dick had called the neurosurgeon, everything had moved so fast, they were in a state of shock.

They were all the more stunned when the surgeon walked into the waiting room and said bluntly, "It's lung cancer. And it looks very, very bad." He talked on, but that was virtually all they heard.

The women broke down crying. "We knew cancer was a possibility," Annette says, "but finding out that way just took us off our feet. We really broke down. It was terrible. The doctor was so blunt! I believe in honesty, but that was cruel."

When Dick regained consciousness in the recovery room, the surgeon came to tell him, "It's malignant. . . . It's not operable. . . . If I were you, I would get my estate in order. . . ."

Dick, too, had difficulty comprehending the news. Cancer seemed impossible—as if the doctor was talking about someone else. "Things like this always happened to some other guy," he says, "not *me*. I had a fine family, we were all very close, a wonderful woman I'd been married to for over thirty years, a successful business; I enjoyed life tremendously. I had too much to live for. I couldn't believe it.

"On top of that, I didn't even know anything about this disease called cancer. At that moment I couldn't remember ever knowing anyone who'd had it, although actually both my uncle and my sister-in-law had passed away from cancer. But my mind was so blown, I couldn't think."

As Dick struggled to clear his mind, he realized that Annette was standing beside his cart. He looked up to see that she, too, had tears in her eyes. Turning to the surgeon, Dick asked, "Is there *anything* I can do?"

The surgeon shrugged. "You could have radiation therapy, but it wouldn't help. It would only make you sick."

"Is there some place else I can *go*?"

The doctor then told Dick he could give him a referral

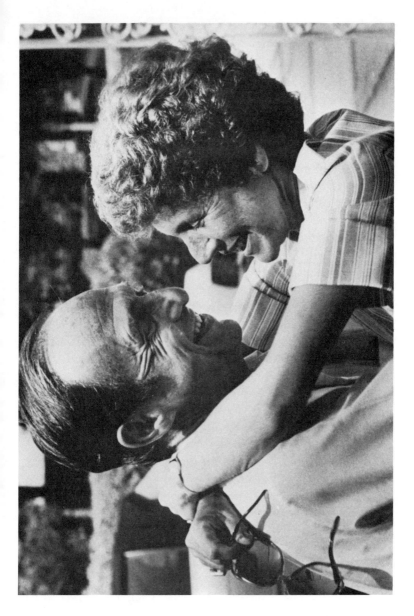

RICHARD AND ANNETTE BLOCH

anywhere else in the country—but that nobody else knew any more.

At this, Dick finally began to cry. Annette reached out and held his hand. She regained her composure first, and held his hand until he stopped crying, too.

Today, far from that initial shock, Dick leans back in his chair and recalls it. "You know, your realization that you have cancer happens faster than an automobile accident. It's terribly sudden. With a car crash, at least you usually have that fraction of a second before you hit. With cancer, you're going along feeling fine, and suddenly," he snaps his fingers, "*cancer*. One word, and you've got it. A lot of people never have any symptoms; or there are people like me, who have symptoms but they feel okay, and they really never think it could be cancer, not for them."

That night, as Dick sat wrestling with despair, a close friend called. Buddy Greenbaum, whose wife had cancer, had gone into action when he heard of Dick's diagnosis. He told Dick that his wife's doctor in Houston was expecting Dick's call that evening. He convinced Dick to make that call even though it was 10:00 at night.

"Come down here tomorrow," the doctor said, after hearing the details. "I'll see you first thing Friday morning."

Dick remembered the words of the surgeon: "If I were you, I would get my estate in order."

"Look," he told the Houston doctor, "I'm dying, I might never get back to Kansas City. I've got a lot of things to wrap up here. Can I see you Monday morning instead?"

Laconically the doctor said, "If you're not here tomorrow, I won't treat you."

That got Dick's attention. "The doctor was telling me that the cancer will never be as treatable as today, and at some point it would become untreatable. What really counted was my life, not some papers on my desk. I went to Houston to save my life.

"What that doctor was saying was, 'This really may be treatable—today.' That had a great deal of impact on me. It also makes sense. I learned later that cancer is never as treatable as it is today, and at some point it's untreatable, period. It's past the turning point."

As Dick and Annette embarked on the Thursday afternoon flight to Houston, Dick wondered whether he would ever see his home again. The doctor's insistence that treatment must begin now was encouraging. But, as the 707 cut through the clouds, Dick was plagued with grim thoughts. It was inoperable, he had been told that. He thought, too, about Annette's sister; on July 1 she had been given at least three months to live—and three days later she died.

Purposefully, he changed his train of thought. He reminded himself of the card his daughter Barbara sent him in 1976. In part it said, "Thank God for your spirit . . . the determination with which you do everything—sometimes bordering on stubbornness!—but displaying a stamina that I must admire. . . . Thank God for your strength." Recalling that message, Dick squeezed Annette's hand and thought, "I *have* to make it. I won't quit. I'll fight it until I beat it."

The following morning Dick registered as an outpatient at M. D. Anderson, bringing with him X rays, slides, and numerous doctors' reports. In an orientation session, he and Annette were shown a film about the renowned institution, where over twelve hundred cancer patients are treated daily, with each case reviewed by a multidisciplinary panel. After his frustrating bouts with individual physicians, Dick was struck by the wisdom of this concept. Annette pointed out, too, the competent, cheerful attitude of the clinic's staff. All told, Dick began to feel he had come to the right place.

Immediately after the orientation, Dick embarked on an exhausting day of tests, including a brain scan, a liver scan, and a painful bone marrow test. At 5:00 P.M., the last test was complete and Dick was told the results would be analyzed over the weekend. Meanwhile, he was free until Monday morning. He and Annette decided to fly to Fort Lauderdale for a peaceful weekend in their apartment.

Annette still recalls that sunny weekend. Dick steered their little speed boat, *After Taxes,* to a tiny isolated island. There they talked about their love for one another, stronger than ever after thirty-one years, three children, and four grandchildren.

As they walked hand in hand down the beach, Annette picked up a stick and drew a heart in the sand. Like a teenager, she wrote their initials in the heart, along with the date, and then, "We Shall Return."

On Monday morning, the Blochs were back in Houston sitting with the doctor to discuss the test results, and the conclusion of M. D. Anderson's panel of doctors. "Dick," the doctor said, "you are a very sick boy. We are going to make you a lot sicker, but we are going to cure you." Then he added, "We are going to cure you so you can work to fight cancer."

Richard Bloch is a man who means what he says. He replied, "If you do, I will."

Five months after he first noticed the pain in his neck and shoulder, Dick was given a treatment plan for his cancer. They had been uncomfortable months, and the five days between the biopsy and this moment had been the worst days of his life. "No matter how bad anything is," he says now, "it can't be as bad as living without hope. Before they even told me what they were going to prescribe for me, I felt I could live with it, as long as I had hope. The wonderful thing is, he wasn't saying, 'We'll *try.*' He was saying I would survive, there was no question about it. We were elated. Those other doctors had just destroyed the quality of my life, because they had taken away my hope of a future. Now we had our first positive ray of hope, and we both felt truly marvelous."

The doctor outlined the therapy tailored to Dick's exact

situation. It would begin with two weeks of radiation therapy. This would kill 72 percent of the cancer cells in his body. (One million of these tiny cells, the doctor explained, could fit on the head of a pin.) The radiation would reduce the cancer to the point where chemotherapy, which is ineffective against a large cancer, could work on the remaining isolated cells. A week's treatment of chemotherapy would also help prevent metastasis, since it would kill any cells that broke off from the main tumor and settled in other parts of the body. Following this, Dick would recuperate for a few weeks, undergo surgery to remove the diseased area, take immunization therapy, and finally be given one year of chemotherapy. By the time he entered the chemotherapy, Dick might be entirely free of cancer; but a recurrence could be fatal, so this preventive treatment was essential.

The next morning Annette and Dick went to the radiation therapy department, where they were led to the section which specializes in therapy on the chest. The walk through the long hallway sent shivers up Dick's spine. On dozens of chairs flanking both sides of the hall, patients sat waiting for treatment, red lines painted on their bald heads and necks, and many of them obviously very ill. To Dick, it was like a scene from Dante's *Inferno*. "My God," he wondered, "is this what they're going to do to me?" In this keyed-up state of mind, he entered a small auditorium. He listened with little comprehension while the radiologist discussed the X rays with about two dozen other physicians. The process was calming; whatever those people in the halls looked like, Dick was getting the help of many experts.

After the brief review, he was taken to another room where he lay on a table under a mock X-ray machine, used to map out future treatments. The radiologist used a computer to determine exact locations and then, with a Magic Marker, placed dots at strategic points on Dick's body, and connected them carefully with a ruler.

"This insures that you get each treatment in exactly the right spot," he explained. While this made sense, Dick couldn't help feeling a little strange, "like one of those sketches for a side of beef—here's the shank, the brisket, the sirloin, and so on." He felt less humorous about all this when he was told not to shower for the next fourteen days, since the markings had to be preserved.

During the next two weeks, Dick had radiation treatments for forty seconds each morning at 8:00, and was then free to do whatever he wanted. The treatments themselves gave him no sensation at all, and he was no longer troubled by the bald and oddly mapped patients in the hallways. "That was because I now understood," he says. "This was strictly a communication problem, and very typical; doctors don't realize what the patient needs to know. Not for the last time, I became aware of a problem almost every cancer patient has: the lack of communication between doctor and patient. Doctors are busy, and they often assume that the patient understands something that, in reality, is a total mystery. If I had known why those patients in the hallway looked like that, I wouldn't have been so frightened.

"This fear of the unknown may lead people to reject a treatment because they're afraid, or they don't understand. But if it is explained so that they know what to expect, then they'll accept it. I've talked with countless other patients, and believe me, this lack of communication is something that 99 patients out of 100 experience."

During these fourteen days Dick and Annette stayed in the Anderson-Mayfair Hotel across the street from the hospital, spending much of their time reading everything they could find about cancer. Through medical reports in magazines and newspapers, they learned about the Simonton Institute (at that time located in Fort Worth, now in Dallas). The Simontons operated on the premise that the mind can stimulate the immune system, and thus help cure cancer, although positive thinking was and is seen as an adjunct to, not a substitute for, traditional medical treatment. With great interest, Dick and Annette noted the documented results of Simonton techniques. Dick decided this could help him, too.

Following a technique the Simontons advocate called "imaging," Dick pictured his cancer as an ugly black mass in his shoulder, "like a glob of tar" which moved and swirled constantly. In his imaging sessions, he repeatedly hit the glob with his fist, so that it broke into little pieces which then dissolved. The image, he felt, worked hand-in-hand with the radiation therapy, which was having the same effect—killing off a percentage of the cells with each treatment.

In the meantime, Annette was interested in what she read about the use of marijuana to relieve nausea in patients who are taking chemotherapy. She and Dick argued about this; he was adamantly opposed to smoking marijuana, and pointed out that, even for cancer patients, its use was still illegal in Texas. Annette was insistent, however, and the night before Dick's first chemotherapy treatment, she and their daughter Nancy baked a batch of marijuana brownies, heavily iced to disguise the taste.

At 7:00 A.M. Dick was taken to one of a dozen beds in a chemotherapy ward. He could not see most of the other patients, whose beds were obscured by privacy curtains—but he could hear "the moans and groans, and the sounds of retching. And the smell! It seemed like a snake pit. When I walked in there that morning and thought about doing this for days, my knees went weak." Dick's time in that ward was to be intensive: during the next week he would take chemotherapy from 7:00 A.M. until at least 7:00 P.M., and sometimes until 11:00 P.M.

In most respects, Dick found M. D. Anderson very good at communicating with the patient. Now, to prepare him for chemotherapy, a nurse patiently and clearly explained just what chemicals he would be receiving, and how they would

be flushed through his system with intravenous saline solution. He felt comforted by this information.

Less comforting was the marijuana brownie Annette had
lovingly urged on him. Just before leaving the hotel, Dick had
braced himself and taken a big bite. "It was the icing that did
me in," he says with a disgusted expression. "She'd made it
terribly rich. I can't imagine any chemotherapy ever being
worse than that icing. I immediately vomited." To this day,
Dick gets queasy at the thought of a brownie, and is quick to
say that he had his first and last experience with marijuana.

There was no doubt after the first day that the chemotherapy was strong stuff. Dick had to be helped to the car so
he could be taken across the street to the hotel. He was not in
the least disheartened by the terrible weakness the chemicals
induced in him. "I was grateful for my sickness," he says. "I
figured if those drugs can make this big strong body of mine
so ill, just think what they're doing to those puny little cancer
cells." This kind of thinking gave Dick and Annette consider-
able comfort during the difficult time to follow.

By the end of the week, Dick was so worn out that he had
to be taken to his plane in a wheelchair. Back in Kansas City,
he stretched out for three weeks of recuperation before his
surgery, fully expecting to feel a little better each day. "Little
did I know!" he says expressively. "I thought I'd have three
weeks of R and R, but instead I got progressively weaker."
Furthermore, Dick's senses of taste and smell had been dis-
torted by the treatments. Even his favorite foods had no ap-
peal; the most carefully made coffee tasted burned to him.
Odors inexplicably bothered him, so that some dried flowers
in his room had to be removed, although he had never before
noticed their smell. The rest of the family went around in
their lightest summer clothes, miserable with the heat, because Dick was so cold that the air conditioner had to be
turned off.

Dick had been warned that he would develop the worst

sore throat of his life exactly fourteen days after his radiation therapy. He did. Searching for a way to describe it, he says, "It was like those charley horses you can get in your leg—but this was in my throat." When it first developed, he could not even swallow water. Once he was able to manage that, Annette tried to tempt him with baby food, and applauded him when he managed a teaspoon of a soft-boiled egg. Dick did his best, knowing that he was losing too much weight. Meanwhile, he kept reminding himself that the therapy must have done a terrific job on the cancer. The doctors, he thought, knew what they were doing; after all, they had predicted this agonizing sore throat with perfect accuracy!

A few days later, the worst was over and Dick was able to swallow some food. Now he was taken by surprise when his hair began to fall out. Of course, he had been prepared for this, and a few stray hairs didn't bother him; but when it came out in large clumps, he was shocked. Within a week, he had no hair anywhere on his body—he had even lost his eyebrows. The surgery was only a week or so away, and five weeks after that his daughter Linda would be getting married. Annette was not taken by Dick's Telly Savalas look, especially not for the wedding, and brought home a toupee, hoping he would be more comfortable in it. He wasn't. After the wedding, he never wore it again, even though it was a full year before his hair was back to normal.

After a rough start, Dick did recuperate and regain his strength. Two nights before the operation, Dick, Annette, and all three daughters arrived in Houston, found the best restaurant in the city, "and had a great night on the town. I remember how all five of us sat on that king-sized bed in the hotel and laughed and giggled. We hugged and kissed each other and laughed some more. Their love gave me great fortitude to face what I was facing."

Just before the surgery, Dick asked one of the attending surgeons how much use of his right arm he would lose. The doctor replied that he did not know. "You're facing the worst kind of surgery," he said. "When we go in, it's not to repair or improve something, it's to remove anything cancerous. You can't come out any better than when you go in, only worse. We're going to get rid of the cancer, wherever we see it. We have no idea how far it's gone. If we have to, we'll take off your shoulder. So you could come out without a right arm."

It took strong pre-operative medication to relax Dick after that.

For the family, the surgery seemed endless. In Dick's room, they paced, or tried to sit still, and although nobody spoke about it, everyone knew there was a possibility they would never see Dick alive again. Their fear accelerated when a nurse came in to tell them the operation was over, and the surgeon wanted to talk to them in the waiting room outside surgery. They waited there for ten minutes before the surgeon appeared.

"Those ten minutes were the most frightening of my entire life," Annette says. "I can't imagine ever having such fear again. I know I was like a caged animal, pacing, praying, talking to myself. I kept telling myself, 'It's going to be all right, it's going to be all right.' Then I would think, 'But what if it isn't?' When the doctor finally came in, I saw his smile, and I almost fainted with relief."

"He's fine," the surgeon said. As the family members wiped away tears of joy, he sat down and explained to them what had occurred in the operation. He had removed the top lobe of Dick's right lung, two ribs and part of a third, as well as certain affected nerves in Dick's right shoulder. The tumor, he said, had shrunk so much that he had been able to remove every trace of it.

The pathology report showed that not one single living cell remained in the tumor—the radiation and chemotherapy had killed the cancer. That meant the surgery was not really necessary. But Dick harbored no resentment about this. "The whole purpose is to get rid of cancer," he says. "Surgery was one of the steps, and it would have been foolish not to do it." As for the odds on Dick's long-term survival, they could not be calculated. To the doctor's knowledge, no lung cancer patient had ever received the same treatment Dick had in the same sequence.

"Every case of cancer is unique," he told Dick, "like a fingerprint. Cancers occur in different ages and backgrounds, with different strengths and weaknesses. This is why statistics about survival are always shaky."

The doctor also explained the consequences of the operation. Because certain nerves in the right shoulder had been removed, Dick's right side would not perspire from now on. He would also lack coordination. "You won't play tennis again," the doctor said.

"Oh yes, I will," Dick said.

Annette enjoys recounting this story. "Dick is such a *determined* person," she says. "I know that once he sets his mind on something, he's going to do it, especially if someone tells him he can't. That challenge is all he needs. The word 'can't' just isn't in his vocabulary. So as soon as they told him he couldn't play tennis, I knew he would."

During the three weeks Dick spent convalescing in the hospital, Annette stayed on at the Anderson-Mayfair, with each one of the Blochs' three daughters in turn spending a week with her. If they had wanted, they could have stayed in Dick's hospital room, where there was an extra sofa bed for family members. Dick was content to be alone at night, but was impressed by M. D. Anderson's policy. "They believe cancer is a family affair. They encourage family togetherness and support."

A few days after his surgery, Dick was put on a regimen of lung exercises. From the first, he was given pain pills, since the doctors believed pain would impede his recovery. And he began the next phase of his program, immunization therapy. This involved a vaccine called BCG, which was administered through a tube in his side directly into the pleural cavity. This vaccine causes an illness similar to tuberculosis, which mobilizes the immune system against a recurrence of lung cancer. Its use in immune therapy is based on the discovery that people who have had tuberculosis rarely contract lung cancer. Within a few days, Dick's temperature hit 105 degrees; then he was given medication for thirty days to cure him of this "TB."

It was not until two weeks after the surgery that Dick fully realized how much use of his right hand and arm he had lost. Far from playing tennis, he was not even able to hold a pencil. A physical therapist was called in, and ran a series of electronic tests to determine the extent of the nerve damage. She then marked a red "X" at eight different points on Dick's right arm and taught Annette how to administer therapy. The therapy was not pleasant. It consisted of touching the eight points in turn with electrodes which sent shocks along the nerves; these shocks would stimulate the nerves to regenerate. "If you've ever shocked yourself," Dick says with a grimace, "you know just how this felt." Twice a day for two and a half hours Annette administered the painful shocks, five seconds at a time, with five second rests between shocks. The reward came on the last day, when the shocks caused Dick's fingers to quiver. The painful therapy was a success.

When Dick walked back in his own front door in Kansas City, he was a changed man. He had weighed 169 pounds six months ago; now he was almost gaunt at 145. He was still hairless, and had a tendency to hold his damaged right arm motionless, to stoop slightly, and to walk with a sliding, shuffling gait. Annette became worried; he seemed to have become an old man. Since her efforts to talk to Dick about it were unproductive, she finally spoke to his doctor. Then she and the doctor sat down and talked to Dick. "After that," he says with a little smile, "I made a real effort to act my age. Stand tall, lift my feet—and smile. (But I was darned if I'd wear that toupee!)"

For the first time in his life, Dick was put on a diet designed to make him gain weight. The combination of chemotherapy, radiation and the sore throat it caused, the surgery, and the lingering memory of the marijuana brownie had killed his appetite. Now, on doctor's orders, he forced himself to take large portions of everything, to eat pancakes floating in syrup and butter, and to down milkshakes. For a man who had fought overweight all his life, it was a strange regimen. Grimly, Dick ate until he reached 155 pounds, which he felt was his ideal weight. The doctor told him to keep going, and it wasn't until he was back at 170 that he was allowed to return to his customary diet.

Then Dick, who had complied with everything until now, suddenly turned into a balky patient. As the time approached to begin twelve months of chemotherapy, one week a month, he announced that he wouldn't do it. He thought he was cured; the tumor had been shown to have no living cancer cells. Moreover, he knew full well how miserable he would be with the chemotherapy. He argued with the doctors: "It may cause problems years from now. Why should I punish my body any further?"

He told the doctor about a woman friend whose lung had been removed the previous year because of cancer, and whose surgeon had denied any need for chemotherapy. Another friend had been diagnosed as having lung cancer just two weeks after Dick was, and his surgeon also maintained that the surgery was sufficient treatment. "My tumor was free of living cancer," Dick argued. "Why don't you give me a clean bill of health?"

As he argued with the doctors at M. D. Anderson, Dick finally found one who disagreed with the chemotherapy program, an intern who said, "Look, Dick, you came through surgery with flying colors. If it was up to me, I wouldn't give you any more chemotherapy. I don't think it's necessary."

"That was all Dick needed to hear," Annette says. "Every other doctor told him to have the chemo, but this was the one he wanted to listen to."

But Dick now felt good enough to be stubborn. "I've made up my mind," he told Annette. "I'm not going to do it."

"Oh yes, you are," she insisted. "You *are* going to take the chemo, if I have to drag you there and hold you down."

"You are going to have chemotherapy," the doctor told him. "It's not debatable."

Reluctantly, Dick assented at last. He was glad he did when, just a few months later, his friend developed cancer in her remaining lung; because she had only one lung, surgery was no longer an option. She died soon thereafter. His second friend lived another two years, until a metastasis to his remaining lung killed him.

Because of these experiences and his reading, Dick feels strongly about follow-up treatment after surgery, and believes that every cancer patient should see an oncologist after surgery, no matter how clean and effective the surgery may seem to be. "Cancer cells are not visible to the naked eye, so there's no way a surgeon can be sure he's removed them all. Moreover, he can't possibly tell whether isolated cancer cells have drifted to another part of the body, to the liver or the brain or the other lung. Chemotherapy is the only way to make sure."

Dick points out that the very word "chemotherapy," like the word "cancer," is loaded with negative implications for many people. "They're scared to death of it, because they've heard so many horror stories. But chemo varies widely; technically speaking, taking an aspirin is chemotherapy. Recently I talked to a woman who had an enormous cancer in her stomach, and was put on a very simple form of chemotherapy, one tablet a day. She took them until she read an article about how terrible chemo is, and then she called her doctor and asked, 'Is this pill what you call chemotherapy?'

"He admitted that it was, and she told him, 'I'm not going to take it anymore. I won't take any chemotherapy. I read it kills people.'"

While patients are often as stubbornly opposed to chemotherapy as Dick initially was, he points out that surgeons, too, sometimes fail to understand the usefulness of this treatment. "I get bitter," he says, hitting the table with his fist, "when I hear about a woman who has a mastectomy, and then her surgeon tells her that's it, she's cured. The cure rate of breast cancer today is about 97 percent—*if* it's treated promptly and correctly, and that means follow-up. That means that after surgery the woman should be sent to an oncologist; let him decide whether chemotherapy is necessary after the surgery.

"The reason follow-up is so important," he adds, "is that in many kinds of cancer, you have only one chance to beat it. Once a kidney has been removed, you can't remove the other one. So you've got to do what you can to prevent metastasis."

A week of chemotherapy every month was the next step of Dick's treatment plan. "It was like a diabolical scheme," Dick says. "Every month they'd let me get well enough so they could make me sick again. It's a strange feeling to walk into the doctor's office feeling good and get treatment that makes you violently sick. It reminded me of having a child who's healthy, and taking him in to get his tonsils out—and of course he's going to feel rotten for a while, and he doesn't understand. But let me add that I once again welcomed this ordeal, because I knew that if it was making me so ill, it had to be killing any remaining cancer cells."

During his first months on chemotherapy, Dick took codeine tablets prescribed for the persistent pain in his shoulder, which was apparently caused by scar tissue from the operation. He tried to stop taking the pills from time to time, only to experience disabling pain. Finally he talked to a doctor at M. D. Anderson, who suggested he meet with a staff psychologist. Dick hesitated—but he went.

The psychologist told Dick a story. "Imagine," he said, "that you are walking across Main Street, but you have a very sore leg. Each step you take causes excruciating pain. You can barely walk; you drag your foot slowly.

"You're in the middle of the street when you look up and see a truck coming at you at sixty miles an hour. What happens? Suddenly you have no pain. You are able to run the rest of the way, to get to safety. The pain doesn't reappear until you're out of danger. What does this prove? The mind is capable of turning off pain if it wants to."

Motivated by this story, Dick went to a psychologist Annette found back in Kansas City who specialized in controlling pain. The psychologist stressed the influence of tension on pain. "I had always thought of myself as a relaxed person," Dick admits, "but I really didn't know the meaning of the word." He was delighted with the deep relaxation the doctor taught him to achieve. Once he was sitting or lying comfortably, he would close his eyes and, beginning with his forehead, tell each part of his body to relax: eyebrows, eyes, nose, mouth, and so on, right down to his toes. When his body was relaxed, he would picture himself floating into an absolutely quiet room. From there he would imagine himself floating into a beautiful garden by a peaceful lake, where the sun streamed through the trees, and he would imagine himself lying in the grass, cradled by the aroma of flowers. The psychologist's prescription—to go through this sequence twice a day—was by far the most pleasant "therapy" Dick had.

The psychologist also asked Dick to think the most beautiful thought he could imagine. Immediately Dick knew what it was: "My wife's love for me."

"Let that love fill your body." Dick felt an amazing sensation of warmth and happiness well through him.

"Now, put your left hand on your chest and push that love into the pain. Push the pain through the shoulder and out."

"It worked!" Dick says, with delight and a little incredulity. Since that day, he has never taken a pain pill. Whenever the shoulder began to hurt, he would recall the sensation of being filled with Annette's love, and force the love into the pain; the pain would vanish. "I could do this anywhere," he adds, "even at a red light, and the pain would be gone before the light changed."

During this time Dick was working on an equally serious result of the surgery—the partial paralysis of his right arm. The man who had boasted that he would play tennis again could not move a finger on his right hand, or lift his arm above his shoulder. He had been warned that he risked permanent atrophy of the muscles unless he began therapy immediately, so as soon as he was home from the hospital, arrangements were made for a physical therapist to come to his home three times a week for an hour each time. Her method was to give him exercises; the first few visits, for instance, she told him to bend the fingers of his right hand, and she would measure his progress. His exercises included moving the arm with weights strapped to it, and raising it in front of a mirror; he practiced religiously every day.

One day when the therapist arrived, Dick had a surprise for her. He was out on the tennis court hitting balls against a backboard. Although he could not yet raise the racket, he could hit a ball that was two or three feet off the ground. Week by week he practiced lifting the racket higher and gripping it more securely. After two months the therapist told Dick he didn't need her any more, and added, "You're one of my outstanding successes." Today Dick has totally regained the use of the muscles in his arm, wrist, and fingers, although he cannot hit the ball as hard as he once did. "My game has never been better, though," he says triumphantly. "I have more control, and I place my shots more accurately."

"It was tougher than he lets on," Annette adds. "Anyone else would have quit. But Dick was determined." As before, tennis is one of Dick's foremost pleasures, and today he plays six times a week.

This diligent work to regain the use of his arm helped Dick weather the difficult year on chemotherapy. He minimized the "few bad days" a month, and lived an otherwise normal life. In July, he and Annette went to Bermuda on business for a week; and in December they spent a month in Acapulco—after Dick's doctor agreed to juggle his chemotherapy treatments slightly.

A great lover of travel, Dick was continually stimulated by these trips Annette insisted they plan. But on a Caribbean cruise over the 1978 Christmas holidays with his three daughters and their husbands, Dick began to feel worse and worse. By the time the ship reached its second port, Grand Cayman, he was so feverish and weak that he called his doctor in Houston, who told him to get to the nearest hospital, have a blood test, and call him with the results.

When he did, the doctor told him to have the test done again and call back; the findings were disturbing. The second test verified the first. "The blood count indicated that I had no resistance to illness at all," Dick recalls. "If I had gotten any kind of infection, I could have died within twenty-four hours. I had to get back to the States immediately." All flights off the island were booked that day, but the doctor made telephone calls until he was able to get seats for Annette and Dick on a flight to Miami.

By coincidence, Dick's oncologist was vacationing in the Miami area; he visited Dick and ordered him to bed, allowing him only to visit the local hospital every other day for blood tests.

One of the blood tests was so bad that the doctor requested verification; the results confirmed the first test. The doctor told Dick he needed a platelet transfusion at M. D. Anderson.

Dick was balky. "I can't believe it's that bad."

"You might not feel that bad, but if you start to bleed anywhere, you won't stop. You're lucky your gums didn't bleed this morning when you brushed your teeth." Still, Dick maintained that he did not want to fly to Houston. Finally the doctor agreed to see what tomorrow's blood test looked like.

As it turned out, even though the bad results had been confirmed, they had been wrong. "Somebody counted the platelets wrong," Dick says, shaking his head. "Oh, the highs and lows of this strange disease!"

By January of 1979 Dick was feeling in top shape. Then, toward the end of the month, he had a scare. He had gone into M. D. Anderson for his routine quarterly examination, expecting to fly on home to Kansas City the next day. But instead of giving Dick the all-clear, the doctor had bad news: a dark mass had shown up on the lung X ray. The diagnostic radiologist and the surgeon agreed that there was a possibility of another tumor. "It could just be scar tissue," the doctor added, "but I want to do a biopsy."

That afternoon, as Dick and Annette sat in the hotel room, he was close to tears. "Just when he thought he was well again, it was back to the operating table," Annette explains. "He was sure he had another tumor. He told me, 'I can't go through it again. I just can't. I quit.'

"I said, 'No, you don't. You have to do this, and you will.'"

The needle biopsy the next day was frustratingly inconclusive. It showed no malignancy, but the Blochs were warned that the needle might have missed the cancerous cells. Dick and Annette would have to live with uncertainty while bi-weekly chest X rays were taken and compared. Amazed to realize cancer could grow so fast that a difference could be seen in two weeks, Dick went for the X rays during the next months religiously. Time after time, they showed no change in the mass. Finally the doctors were satisfied that it was scar tissue, not cancer.

At the end of March, the Blochs again returned to Houston for Dick's routine examination. After the test results were in, the doctor examined Dick and told him, "You won't be taking any more chemotherapy treatments."

"Those," Dick says, beaming, "were the most beautiful words I'd ever heard."

A year later, however, he heard more beautiful words, when he returned to Houston for his semi-annual checkup in May 1980. It had been two years since his surgery. After the examination, the doctor said, "Dick, I won't be seeing you anymore."

Dick was surprised. "What?"

"We consider you cured." He went on to explain that with Dick's type of cancer, a patient who is cancer-free for two years has no more chance of cancer than the man on the street. (This time period, Dick cautions, varies according to the type of cancer.)

"I couldn't believe it at first," Dick says. "I never thought I would hear that word—'cured.' There surely is a good Lord above!"

On the flight back to Kansas City, Dick Bloch sat and tried to realize that he was no longer a cancer patient. He was overwhelmed with joy. Annette, beside him, was glowing.

"Remember what the doctor at M. D. Anderson told me, two years ago?" Dick asked her. "He said, 'We are going to cure you so you can work to fight cancer.' Well, they kept their word—and I'm going to keep mine." At that moment, Richard Bloch made a commitment to devote the rest of his life to helping cancer patients.

"God works in mysterious ways," Annette says. "I believe Dick became ill for a reason. He was a brilliant man, still young, in his early fifties, and semiretired—he was too vital and capable to be unproductive. Perhaps God made him sick and better again so he would realize what cancer was, and devote himself to fighting it."

Back home again, Dick considered what he knew about the fight against cancer. His knowledge wasn't medical or theoretical, like a doctor's or a researcher's; it was personal. He knew how he felt, and he knew how some of his fellow patients had felt. "I learned I wasn't unique—that most people had the same reactions I had. I regretted, though, that I never had the chance to speak to someone else who had recovered from lung cancer. That might really have helped me—helped me see that recovery really was possible." From that thought came the idea for the Cancer Hotline.

The concept of the Hotline was that volunteers who had experienced cancer could help cancer patients, particularly patients who had just received their diagnoses and didn't know where to turn. Dick set up the first Hotline in Kansas City. It operates without funding, using office space provided by H & R Block and brochures printed free of charge by local printers and distributed at no cost (for instance, in the statements sent out by the utility companies).

Hotline calls go into an existing crisis intervention telephone service, and are relayed immediately to trained volunteers; one goal of the service is that every caller should be called back within fifteen minutes. The volunteers, interestingly enough, are not taught what to say so much as they are taught what *not* to say during these conversations.

"I didn't think extensive training was necessary," Dick explains. "If the caller wants to talk to someone with formal education, let him call his doctor." In terms of dispensing information, the volunteer is likely to recommend four important steps to each caller: get prompt treatment; get proper treatment (which means a second opinion, and a consultation with an oncologist); get thorough treatment (follow the doctor's advice); and read the book *Getting Well Again,* by Carl and Stephanie Simonton (the book Dick used in developing imagery techniques to fight his own cancer).

What do you *not* say to a cancer patient? Volunteers are taught not to "tell their war stories," since no two cancers are alike. They are also told not to give false reassurances, such as "You're going to make it," since this destroys credibility with the patient. What volunteers *can* do is share the feelings they have had as cancer patients. They also tell patients how to seek proper medical advice, and what rights to retain. Dick gives a sample conversation, in which a woman calls in who has a lump on her breast; the doctor wants to take a biopsy.

"What should I do?" she asks, half-frantic.

"Go ahead and get the biopsy, right away."

"But I don't want a radical mastectomy!"

"Then don't give him permission to do a mastectomy—just to do a biopsy and examine the lymph glands."

"Are you sure?"

"Yes. Once you get the results of the biopsy, then you have the information you need to figure out your options."

The Kansas City Hotline has been so successful that a survey of callers indicated that an amazing 99 percent felt satisfied with the help they got when they called. As a result, hotlines patterned after this one are being established in several other cities.

At the same time as he was working on the Hotline, Dick was also putting together a second unique service, based on the multidisciplinary approach at M. D. Anderson. This project, the Cancer Treatment Panel, brought together specialists in various medical disciplines to review individual cases as a group and suggest treatment plans.

"You see," Dick says, "I realized that many, many people are unable to go to a major cancer center for one reason or another. But they are still entitled to a chance at life. Now, every town of any size has all kinds of medical specialists; it's just a question of getting them together so that their group expertise is available."

To the creation of the panel, Dick brought all the organizational skills and determination he had used to help build H & R Block into a successful national company. He met with oncologists, cancer surgeons, radiologists, and numerous other specialists; on September 2, 1980, the Cancer Treatment Panel became a reality, with dozens of doctors signed up to work on a rotating basis. Once a week a panel of five specialists— medical oncologist, surgeon, radiologist, pathologist, and psychiatrist or psychologist—convened to review up to four cases, going over the patients' medical records, X rays, reports, slides, and any other available information. The panel would review the treatment plan the patient's doctor had proposed and approve it or recommend alternatives. These recommendations were discussed in the patient's presence, and then written down and sent to both the referring doctor and the patient.

The open discussions in the presence of patients and their relatives was unique in the medical world. While the group medical advice was undeniably the most important feature of this plan, Dick found in talking to patients that as a side effect the panel also gave them a markedly improved sense of confidence and hope. What did this service cost? Dick smiles. "Nothing. Everyone volunteered their services. The patient got the review for free."

The Cancer Treatment Panel was so successful that Dick decided to expand the concept. At the end of April 1982, the panel was terminated; on May 1, the R. A. Bloch Cancer Management Center opened its door. The nonprofit center is basically a more sophisticated version of the panel, and is staffed by doctors who are expert in narrow specializations; one of its panels, for instance, includes six doctors from different disciplines who specialize in treating breast cancer. "Believe me," Dick says, "these guys are so darn technical you wouldn't believe it. They'll talk about the exact location of a lump and what significance that has. In all modesty, there's nothing like this anywhere else."

The Cancer Management Center, like the Cancer Treatment Panel, is for everyone, and the review is free to patients who can't afford to pay for it. For others, the cost is $500, to cover the consulting fees paid to the doctors.

The center recommends only established therapies. When appropriate, a patient is directed to a specific institution which specializes in treating his or her form of cancer; a leukemia patient, for instance, will be told about Fred Hutchins Hospital in Seattle.

The center has received a great deal of publicity since it began, and interested people around the country have called Dick and Annette to talk about building on this concept in their communities. Needless to say, the Blochs are very receptive to these inquiries. "Someday, we'd like to see these centers in every major city in the country," Dick says.

Dick has another dream, equally broad in scope: a program called PDQ. The letters stand for Protocol, Delivery, Query, and the program will be a nationwide computer linkup formed in conjunction with the National Cancer Institute in Bethesda, Maryland.

"I got to thinking about all the little towns and cities that don't have cancer centers, maybe don't even have specialists," Dick says. "What can be done for those people?"

What can be done, according to Dick's dream, is to program a computer with all known treatments for the various types of cancer. "Then, suppose there's a doctor in Podunk, North Dakota. He's got a computer terminal, and he's on our system. He picks up the phone and tells the computer, 'I've got a case of cancer number 65, in location A5' (that's the area of the body) 'on a man who's forty-four years old. He's got a history of diabetes, and he's deaf in his left ear. How do I treat him?'

"And then," Dick lights up with enthusiasm, "the computer just rattles out the answers. 'Memorial Sloan-Kettering recommends the following protocols . . . The University of Southern California recommends the following protocols . . .' It's fantastic. *And* it gives him other relevant information, like 'Caution: Patient's history of diabetes means there may be a reaction to drug so-and-so.' It will tell him the usual response time to the treatment, the side effects, everything. So here's a guy in a little town, without access to the big cancer centers, and he knows the very latest and best treatment for his patient— at a cost of $10. And during the next year the computer will call him back any time there's an improvement or change in that treatment plan."

In keeping his vow to fight cancer, Richard Bloch has come up with projects of breathtaking scope. Even Annette is sometimes awed by the grandeur of his ideas. But then, they are also just what she expects from him. She explains, "Dick has tackled this just as he would a new business. It's the same kind of commitment. His mind is always moving on this, how he can help cancer patients, and it's a commitment we share. We feel we have a tremendous debt to pay—he was very fortunate—and we intend to pay it."

Dick has not accomplished what he wants to; PDQ is not yet a reality. When it is, there will be more projects, beyond a doubt. Even so, he doesn't really feel he has done so much. "I have a limited goal," he says earnestly. "I just want to help the next human being who has cancer."

PUBLISHER'S AFTERWORD

All twelve people profiled in this book are doing well. The publisher regrets to announce, however, that the inspiration for this book—Bobbie Shook, the author's wife—died May 4, 1983.

DATE DUE		
FEB 24 84 RETURNED DEC 15 85		
88		MAR 24 2011
FEB 10 1989 OCT 0 8 1993		
Returned NOV 12 1998		
Returned DEC 1 0 2003 NOV 1 2 2005		